D0313964

ANDERSONIAN LIBRARY
★
WITHDRAWN
FROM
LIBRARY
STOCK
★
UNIVERSITY OF STRATHCLYDE

Ophthalmic Anaesthesia

**Books are to be returned on or before
the last date below.**

LIBREX—

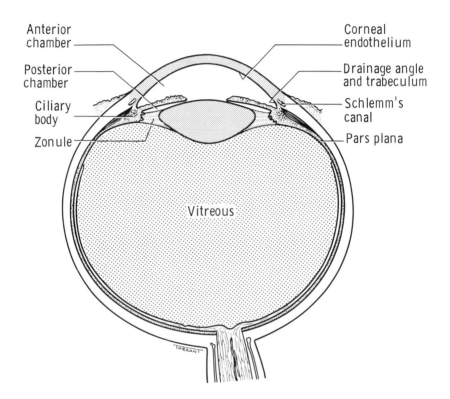

Anterior chamber

Posterior chamber

Ciliary body

Zonule

Corneal endothelium

Drainage angle and trabeculum

Schlemm's canal

Pars plana

Vitreous

TARRANT

Frontispiece An antero-posterior section of the globe of the eye.

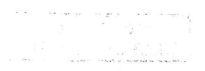

#11157199

Ophthalmic Anaesthesia

G. Barry Smith TD, DA, FFARCS (Eng)

Director of Anaesthesia, Moorfields Eye Hospital, London;
Honorary Clinical Teacher, Institute of Ophthalmology,
University of London; Honorary Clinical Assistant,
Maxillo-Facial Unit, Queen Victoria Hospital, East Grinstead

Edward Arnold

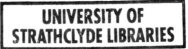

UNIVERSITY OF
STRATHCLYDE LIBRARIES

© G. Barry Smith 1983

First published 1983
by Edward Arnold (Publishers) Ltd
41 Bedford Square, London WC1B 3DQ

British Library Cataloguing in Publication Data
Smith, G. Barry
   Ophthalmic anaesthesia.
   1. Anesthesia in ophthalmology
   I. Title
   617′.96751   RF52

   ISBN 0 7131 4339 1

All Rights Reserved. No part of this publication may be reproduced, stored in a retrieval system, or transmitted in any form or by any means, electronic, mechanical, photocopying, recording or otherwise, without the prior permission of Edward Arnold (Publishers) Ltd.

Whilst the advice and information in this book are believed to be true and accurate at the date of going to press, neither the author nor the publisher can accept any legal responsibility or liability for any errors or omissions that may be made.

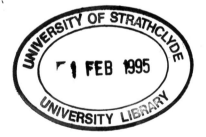

UNIVERSITY OF STRATHCLYDE
1 FEB 1995
UNIVERSITY LIBRARY

Filmset in 10/11pt Compugraphic Times by
CK Typesetters Ltd., 26 Mulgrave Road, Sutton, Surrey
Printed in Great Britain by Spottiswoode Ballantyne Ltd,
Colchester and London

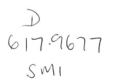

D
617.9677
SMI

Preface

Until recently, ophthalmic anaesthesia has been somewhat neglected as, whenever the anaesthetist lacked the necessary skill, or the patient had some major concurrent disease, the surgeon would opt to perform the operation under local anaesthesia.

The last few years have provided the eye surgeon with new instrumentation and this has made the operation both more complex and more time consuming.

Even frail, sick and elderly patients need to be unconscious for considerable periods and the new breed of ophthalmic surgeon understands and requires precise physiological conditions to control the intraocular pressure, the volume of the contents of the eye, the blood sugar or haemorrhage in the surgical field to achieve his surgical objective. It is to meet this challenge that this book has been produced, to encourage an interest in a changing field of anaesthesia.

1983   GBS

Acknowledgements

I wish to express my grateful thanks to my consultant colleagues at Moorfields Eye Hospital without whose help this book would not have been written. My gratitude is extended to the Dean and to the Institute of Ophthalmology for some of the illustrations.

The graphs on pages 2 and 3 were redrawn from a paper entitled 'Intraocular and intracranial pressure during respiratory alkalosis and acidosis' by R.B. Smith, A.A. Aass and E.M. Nemoto in the *British Journal of Anaesthesia 1981*, **53,** 967.

Special mention must be made of the beautiful ultrasonogram which has been given to me by that leading medical physicist, Dr Marie Restori. She provides an invaluable service to ophthalmology by not only displaying the structure of the eye in health and disease with ultrasound, but also making the use of this new diagnostic tool comprehensible to those without knowledge of this growing specialty.

Quite a lot of surgical ophthalmology has rubbed off onto me during the last fifteen years particularly from Lorimer Fison, John Wright, Dave McLeod, Rolph Blach, Dick Welham and Bob Cooling. If I have accidently misunderstood their teaching, I apologize.

Mrs Marion Lynn tactfully improved the grammar and punctuation while she typed the manuscript.

Lastly, and not least, I thank my devoted wife, Lynn, for putting up with me and with this book.

Contents

1

The intraocular pressure and anaesthesia

Definition

Intraocular pressure (IOP) is the tension exerted by the contents of the globe on the corneoscleral envelope.

The corneoscleral envelope is inelastic and the pressure is related to the volume of the contents, the two main variables of which are the aqueous humour and the rich network of blood vessels which line the inside of the eye, particularly in the choroid. Very small changes in volume lead to major changes in pressure; while operations which indent or deform the envelope cause equally large changes in pressure. This description of the pressure–volume relationship is only an approximation which is sufficiently accurate for the practical anaesthetist. The distensibility of cornea and sclera has been measured by Gloster *et al.* (1957) and more recently by Woo *et al.* (1972). It is often forgotten that the IOP of a perforated or incised eye is atmospheric, and when surgeons talk of raised pressure during a cataract extraction, they are in fact talking about a change in the volume of the contents of the globe relative to the envelope. The blood vessels of the choroid constitute a large and variable volume in the eye. They behave in a similar manner to intracranial vessels and constrict during hypocapnia produced by hyperventilation. This effect has been elegantly demonstrated by R.B. Smith in a graphical form, as may be seen in Figs 1.1 and 1.2.

The retina is very sensitive to hypoxia and it is easy to enumerate conditions in anaesthetic practice in which the IOP could be higher than the systolic blood pressure (BP), thereby preventing perfusion of the retina. If this situation is sustained for several minutes, ischaemia resulting in blindness may occur.

Normal intraocular pressure

The normal IOP is 12–16 mmHg in the erect posture and 2–3 mmHg higher when lying down. It is kept remarkably constant by a dynamic balance between the production and drainage of aqueous humour. It is reduced in total body dehydration using glycerol, but osmotic agents

1

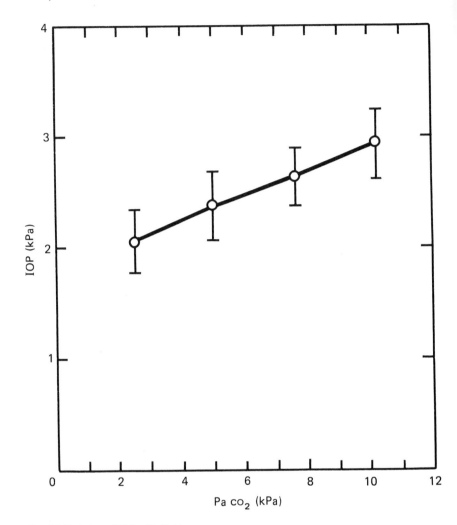

Fig. 1.1 Variation of IOP with Pa_{CO_2}.

such as mannitol have a disappointing effect as the vitreous is avascular and the marked increase in circulatory volume congests the highly vascular choroid coat of the eye.

Everyday fluctuations in blood pressure have little effect on IOP but induced hypotension may cause the pressure to fall to atmospheric, while sustained systemic hypertension is often reflected in a raised IOP. Coughing and other Valsalva-like manoeuvres produce a marked, but short-lived, rise in pressure.

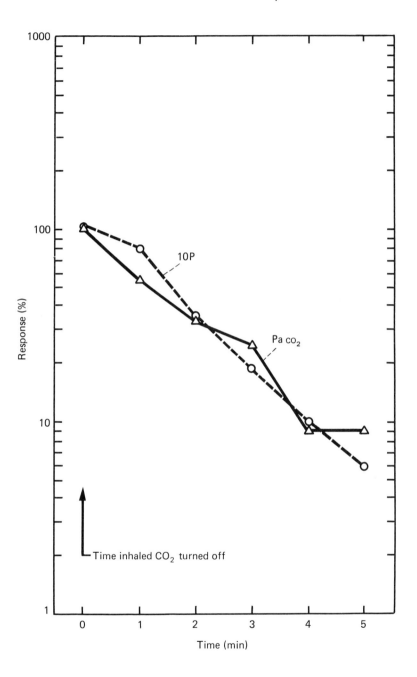

Fig. 1.2 Per cent total response during rapid washout of carbon dioxide.

There is a tendency for IOP to return to normal values very rapidly and it was once the custom among some surgeons to press firmly on the globe for a minute or two, prior to cataract extraction. This had the effect of expelling aqueous through the trabeculum in the angle and when the pressure was removed, the IOP was much reduced. Various devices to achieve a similar result are still in use in some centres. However, the effect is momentary and the capacity of the ciliary body to produce aqueous is so large that the value of this procedure in modern surgical practice is discounted in many centres.

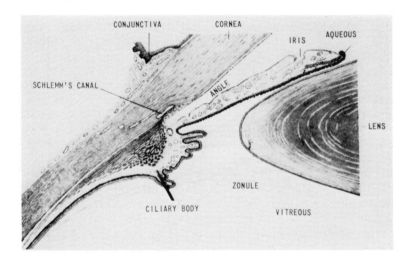

Fig. 1.3 Cross-section of the ciliary body and drainage angle of the eye.

Features of the anatomy and physiology of aqueous humour

Aqueous humour maintains IOP and the spherical form of the globe. It is a major transport system in the eye for oxygen, glucose, proteins and inflammatory cells as well as drugs. It plays an important part in the nourishment of the lens and the endothelium which lines the inner surface of the cornea. The endothelium is a metabolically active layer controlling the water content of the cornea and, thus, its transparency. It obtains about half its oxygen requirement by direct diffusion through the cornea and the remainder from the aqueous.

Systemically administered drugs enter the eye with the aqueous but there is a distinct barrier preventing drugs of high molecular weight passing from the blood into the aqueous. Drugs instilled into the conjunctival sac enter the aqueous of the anterior chamber of the eye very rapidly under the influence of the cellular pumping action of the endothelium. Unfortunately, this applies to noxious substances such as acids and ammonia as well as therapeutic substances and may lead to rapid blindness as the result of accident, therapeutic mishap or assault. All drugs given by the conjunctival route should be carefully buffered to give a neutral reaction.

Aqueous humour is formed by the ciliary body which is a vascular part of the uveal tract situated in front of the pars plana and behind the attachment of the fibres of the suspensory ligament of the lens. The ciliary body has its surface area increased by being thrown into about eighty folds, each 2–3 mm high, called ciliary processes. These are richly supplied by a vascular plexus and covered by an epithelium which is two cells deep. The surface layer of cells is non-pigmented and appears to be an impervious, continuous layer; that is, it is impervious to proteins and substances of high molecular weight but apparently allows electrolytes to pass freely. Aqueous humour is not, however, a simple protein-free filtrate of blood plasma, since it contains a high concentration of ascorbic acid, a low concentration of glucose and a small but constant concentration of all the proteins found in blood.

Macri (1980) has demonstrated that the permeability of the ciliary epithelium can be changed radically in a few moments under the influence of prostaglandins and then produces a 'secondary aqueous' rich in proteins and fibrinogen, the trigger being any major change or trauma to the eye, such as cataract extraction.

The circulation of aqueous humour

The majority of aqueous flows forward through the fibres of the suspensory ligament of the lens and then through the narrow slit between the anterior capsule of the lens and the posterior surface of the iris and gains the anterior chamber through the pupil. It then flows laterally to the angle of the anterior chamber where it enters the meshwork of the trabeculum and runs into the circular canal of Schlemm. Communications between the canal and the episcleral veins allow the aqueous to return to the venous system. This drainage of aqueous is essentially a passive process, but the capacity of the trabecular meshwork can be altered by the pull of the muscular fibres in the iris and the ciliary muscle which tend to open the trabecular spaces.

About a third of the aqueous produced is reabsorbed through the veins of the iris and choroid. A number of drugs influence the production and drainage of aqueous and thus the IOP. The action of some of these drugs is summarized in Table 1.1.

Table 1.1 Action of drugs on IOP

	Dose	IOP
Anxiolytics, premedicants, analgesics		
Diazepam (Al Abrack)	10 mg i.v.	Reduced
Fluritrazepam (Lauret)	0.015–0.03 mg/kg i.v.	Reduced
Droperidol (Smith)	5–10 mg i.v.	Reduced
Haloperidol (Eyada)	0.5 mg i.v.	Reduced by 15%
Chlorpromazine (Couada)		Reduced by 20–30%
Atropine (Schwartz)	0.4–1.0 mg i.m.	No change
Scopolamine (Schwartz)	0.4 mg i.m.	No change
Morphine (Duncalf)	8–15 mg i.m.	Reduced
Fentanyl (Eyada)	0.05–0.1 mg i.m.	Reduced by 20% with controlled ventilation
Phenoperidine (Steele)	0.5–1.0 mg i.v.	Reduced
Induction agents		
Thiopentone (Couadau)	2.5 mg/kg i.v.	Reduced by 30%
Methohexitone (Eichelbauer)	6 mg/kg	Reduced
Etomidate (Oji)	0.3 mg/kg	Reduced by 5.1 mmHg
Althesin (Fordham)		Reduced by 4–10 mmHg
Propanidid (Pelcoldowa)	10 mg/kg i.v.	No change
Ketamine (Duncalf)	1–2 mg/kg i.v.	Raised
(Ausinsch)	5 mg i.m.	Raised by 0.5–2 mmHg
Neuromuscular agents		
Suxamethonium* (Duncalf)	1 mg/kg	Raised (see text)
Decamethonium* (Duncalf)	0.3 mg/kg	Raised
All curare-like agents*		Reduced pressure with ventilation
Gases		
Nitrous oxide		No effect except in the presence of intraocular gas
Cyclopropane		Variable effect probably related to depression of respiration
Volatile agents		
Ether (Komblueth)		Initially slightly elevated but reduced in Stage 3 Plane 3
Chloroform (Magora)		Reduced
Trichlorethylene (Adams)	0.4%	Pressure reduced if ventilated
(other authors)	—	Pressure raised
Halothane (Runciman)	0.5%	Pressure reduced by 5 mmHg but by more in glaucoma or if combined with ventilation
Enflurane (Runciman)	1%	Reduced by 40% with controlled respiration and normocapnia
Isoflurane (Ausirisch)		Reduced by 2 mmHg
Methoxyflurane (Ivankovic)		Reduced in proportion to concentration

*Laryngoscopy and endotracheal intubation raise the IOP in most patients.

Pathology

Disturbances of the circulation of aqueous humour may cause raised IOP (called glaucoma) or lowered IOP (called phthisis). The former condition is common in the elderly. Excessive production of aqueous is rarely a problem and tends to occur only in certain congenital vascular anomalies and in conditions in which the vascularity of the iris is increased, such as rubeosis which may occur in diabetes and some other diseases influencing the vascularity of the eye.

The more common types of glaucoma result from an obstruction to the outflow of aqueous.

Chronic glaucoma

Chronic simple glaucoma has an increasing incidence with age, and sometimes a family history is obtained. The onset is insidious and peripheral vision is lost in the early stages. The drainage angle of the eye is open and the trabeculum appears normal but is not acting efficiently. Medical treatment over long periods aims to stabilize the condition. Pilocarpine, eserine and ecothiopate drops constrict the pupil, pull on the trabecular meshwork and open up the spaces. Adrenaline drops and acetazolamide tend to reduce the production of aqueous humour by the ciliary body. Recently beta-blockers such as timolol have been used in increasing quantities as eyedrops. These have the effect of reducing IOP without constricting the pupil, but they may cause systemic effects such as bronchoconstriction.

The anaesthetic implicaions of these various types of treatment cannot be ignored. The drugs acting on the pupil obscure this valuable sign of anaesthesia for weeks; while ecothiopate causes such a decrease in plasma cholinesterase that serious prolongation of the actions of suxamethonium and the 'ester' local anaesthetics, such as procaine, is likely to occur. Occasionally, systemic symptoms such an abdominal pain and diarrhoea lead to false diagnoses. Adrenaline drops lead to red eyes mimicking conjunctivitis. Acetazolamide, apart from its diuretic properties, not infrequently causes dyspesia and skin rashes. There are a number of patients in whom it seems to have caused acute yellow atrophy of the liver even when no general anaesthetic has been given.

Failure to achieve adequate medical control is an indication for surgical drainage of aqueous from the anterior chamber. Many procedures have been attempted to produce drainage of aqueous into a subconjunctival bleb from which it will be absorbed. At present, a trabeculectomy is frequently performed in which a segment of trabecular meshwork is excised under a scleral flap. The anaesthetic management is aimed at producing a relaxed patient but not great depression of IOP as it is important to retain sufficient rigidity of the globe for the dissection of the scleral flap and also a slight expulsive force to enable an iridectomy to be done through the trabeculectomy without damaging the lens.

Acute glaucoma

In this condition, the iris occludes the drainage angle. There is often a combination of precipitating factors such as a narrow anatomical angle, a pupil dilated by darkness or atropine-like drugs, an iris ballooned forward by a collection of fluid unable to escape through the pupil (iris bombé), or an iris pressed forward by a swollen cataractous lens. There is frequently a history of cough or recent respiratory tract infection.

The acute phase is associated with loss of vision, pain and haloes often attended by surgical shock and vagal symptoms of vomiting and abdominal pain. The cornea is cloudy and IOP is extremely high, 50-60 mmHg.

Medical treatment with intensive meiosis and dehydration with oral glycerol and acetazolamide usually brings the IOP back to a safe level and allows planned surgery to take place in a few days.

The anaesthetic management is not easy. The patient, who is frequently elderly, has been rendered very depleted of water and electrolytes by the initial vomiting and the subsequent dehydration therapy; he often has a residual chest infection; and he may have eaten very little since the onset of the acute phase. The eye, although 'safe' in the ophthalmological sense, often has a tension of 30 mmHg, and sudden decompression of the globe should be avoided to reduce the risk of choroidal haemorrhage. There is the additional problem that a narrow angle in the other eye may induce the surgeon either to perform a bilateral procedure or to request anaesthesia within a few days to perform a prophylactic iridectomy on the second eye.

There is considerable merit in giving a halothane anaesthetic for the first eye, which will reduce IOP satisfactorily, and in recommending the use of local anaesthesia for the second eye. If a general anaesthetic is required, then halothane should be avoided and enflurane substituted.

The value of etomidate as an aid to general anaesthesia in acute glaucoma has recently been shown by Oji and Holdcroft (1979). The intraocular pressure falls rapidly following induction with a dose of 10 mg/kg body weight and remains low for an hour or two. The cause of this fall has not been explained.

Congenital glaucoma or buphthalmos

Although rare, this condition does present, usually soon after birth, with enlarged cloudy corneas and photophobia. When unilateral, it is associated with the Sturge-Weber syndrome and the affected side of the body is covered with capillary naevi.

The ophthalmic surgeon is interested in obtaining a baseline from which to measure IOP so that repeated measurements over weeks, months and years will record the benefits of treatment. Until ten years ago, ether anaesthesia was the only acceptable method of obtaining this base, as, unlike all other anaesthetics, its effect on IOP was minimal with a tendency to cause a small reduction of IOP.

The introduction of intramuscular ketamine in 1965 was followed by its use for the monitoring of IOP by Marynen and Libert (1976); Anatal (1978). In the author's experience, a high intramuscular dose produces the most satisfactory and reproducible results. This dose may raise IOP a little but not as much as a similar intravenous dose. The surgical management of this condition is to create a drainage cleft in the drainage angle of the eye by performing a goniotomy. The conditions produced by ketamine are inadequate for this delicate operation to be performed under an operating microscope owing to grimacing, sighing and yawning. It is therefore necessary to change from ketamine to a formal endotracheal anaesthetic. This transition is frequently associated with problems in a neonate with an immature respiratory centre. It seems, at present, easier to use light halothane or enflurane for a short time rather than resort to curarization.

Measurement of intraocular pressure

While invasive monitoring of pressures within body spaces has become an everyday procedure for anaesthetists, it has not yet become so for IOP, partly because of the delicacy of the eye, partly because of the dangers of introducing infection, and partly because very small changes in the volume of the aqueous produce major pressure changes. It remains a research tool principally for use in animal experiments.

Historically, IOP has been measured by the Schiotz (1920) or indentation technique in which a small plunger activated by a weight and acting through simple levers indents the anaesthetized cornea. (Fig 1.4 shows this instrument in use). A simple pointer on an arbitrary scale shows a reading which can be read off on a nomogram against the weights used. A more elegant and, in expert hands, more accurate method is the Perkins (1965) version of the Goldmann applanation tonometer (shown in Fig 1.5) in which a transparent plunger flattens the previously flaresceined cornea. The observer exerts graduated pressures through a milled wheel and tries to match the observed ends of an illuminated, engraved pattern as seen through the eyepiece.

Both techniques are simple, portable, non-invasive and can be used on the supine patient with either local or general anaesthesia. The Schiotz instrument suffers from considerable inaccuracies from the friction of its moving parts, and repeated readings become progressively lower as

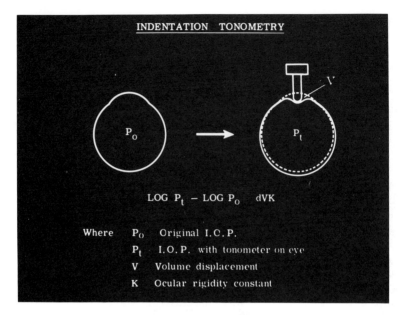

INDENTATION   TONOMETRY

$$\text{LOG } P_t - \text{LOG } P_0 \quad dVK$$

Where P_0 Original I.O.P.

P_t I.O.P. with tonometer on eye

V   Volume displacement

K   Ocular rigidity constant

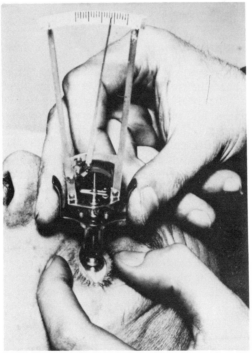

Fig. 1.4 Indentation tonometry using a Schiotz tonometer.

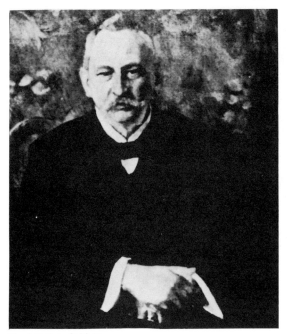

Fig. 1.5 H.J. Schiotz.

aqueous is squeezed out of the eye. The readings from either instrument include a value for the rigidity of the cornea, which may vary from patient to patient.

It is a simple matter to monitor IOP before and during many types of surgery but it is not easy to monitor IOP during the immediate postoperative period after eye surgery, when it would be extremely interesting and perhaps valuable in clinical management. It is not uncommon, after cataract surgery with a completely watertight section closed by many fine sutures, for the IOP to be raised at the first dressing 24 hours postoperatively. Similarly, many scleral indentation procedures for retinal detachment leave the patient with a hard eye, creating an iatrogenic type of acute glaucoma with its associated symptoms of pain and vomiting.

References

Antal, M. (1978). Ketamine anaesthesia and intraocular pressure. *Annals of Ophthalmology* **10** (9), 1281, 1289.
Friedenwald, J.S. (1957). Tonometer calibration: an attempt to remove the discrepancies found in the 1954 calibration used for Schiotz tonometers.

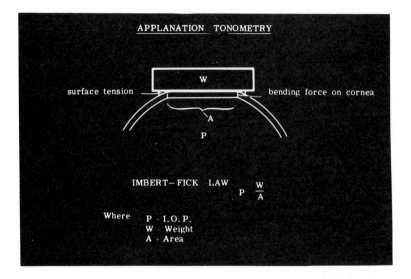

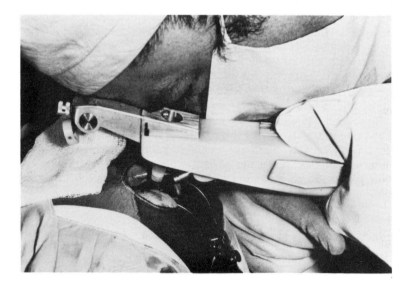

Fig. 1.6 Perkins applanation tonometer.

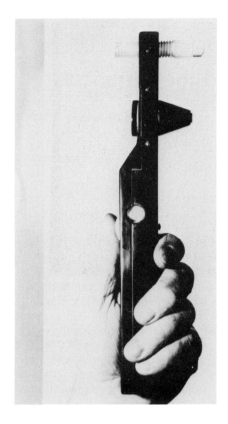

Fig. 1.7 Perkins applanation tonometer.

Transactions of the American Academy of Ophthalmology and Otolaryngology **61**, 108.

Gloster, J., Perkins, E.S. and Pommier, M. (1957). Extensibility of strips of sclera and cornea. *British Journal of Opthalmology* **41**, 103.

Macri, F.J. (1980). The effects of prostaglandins on aqueous humour dynamics. *Prostaglandins* **20**(2), 179.

Marynen, L. and Libert (1976). Ocular tonometry in the child under general anaesthesia with IM Ketamine. *Acta anaesthesiologica belgica* **27** Suppl., 29.

Oji, E.O. and Holdcroft, E. (1979). The ocular effects of etomidate. *Anaesthesia* **34**(3), 245.

Perkins, E.S. (1965). Hand held tonometer. *British Journal of Ophthalmology* **49**, 191.

Shiotz, H.J. (1920). Tonometry. *British Journal of Ophthalmology* **4**, 201.

Woo, S,. Kobagashi, A.S., Schlegal, W.A. and Lawrence, C. (1972). Non-linear material properties of intact cornea and sclera. *Experimental Eye Research* **14**, 29.

2

Muscle relaxants and the extraocular muscles

Gross anatomy and physiology

The four rectus muscles and the two obliques comprise the extraocular muscles (EOMs). The detailed actions of these muscles are of immediate interest to anatomists, neurologists and ophthalmologists, rather than anaesthetists, and the reader seeking detailed information should consult *Eugene Wolff's Anatomy of the Eye and Orbit* (Last, 1968) or Davson's (1980) *The Physiology of the Eye.*

There is no doubt that the levator of the upper lid which is supplied by the third (oculomotor) nerve is an anatomical member of the EOMs. The eye is also influenced by the facial muscles, particularly the orbicularis oculi, contraction of which causes 'squeezing'. The orbit contains smooth muscle which is diffusely distributed; there is a condensation of this in a thin sheet beneath the tendon to the levator of the upper lid, called Müller's muscle.

The EOMs hold the globe like a walnut in a nutcracker and an increase in muscular tension not only squeezes the globe but retracts it against the orbital fat pad. This raises intraocular tension. Although deep planes of anaesthesia or heavy curarization was once advocated to control the simultaneous contraction of opposing muscles, there is little evidence that muscular tension is a major problem in most operations even when the patient is lightly anaesthetized or minimally curarized. Adequate relaxation of the muscles produces a fixed, central pupil. In lighter planes, the eye turns upward as in sleep (Bell's phenomenon) and the cornea is protected by the upper lid. This movement of the globe, caused by the superior rectus muscle, is inconvenient for the surgeon, who usually wishes to work in the upper part of the eye. To obtain the correct position, a traction suture is passed under the insertion of the superior rectus tendon. The traction on the superior rectus to depress the globe forcibly may send this muscle into visible spasm. Anaesthesia should be sufficiently deep to relax this spasm and in addition the surgeon normally relaxes some of the tension on this muscle before attempting any difficult intraocular manipulation.

Physiology of the extraocular muscles

Eye movements are under the control of co-ordinating centres situated in the occipital cortex and the superior colliculi from which impulses pass to the motor centres in the tegmentum, pons and medulla. The motor neurons in these centres fire at a rate of 100 impulses per second, but this can rise above 300 impulses per second. Each axon of the nerve supplies a motor unit of only about six muscle fibres (compared with over 100 in a typical skeletal muscle).

In 1963, Hess and Pilar described two types of muscle fibre in the EOM of the cat—twitch fibres and tonic fibres. This finding has since been confirmed in man by Katz and Eakins, 1969.

The fast, white, twitch fibres have a pattern of regularly arranged fibrils. On electron microscopy these form complex, regular, longitudinal and transverse arrangements called triads which are presumed to permit the rapid transmission of impulses throughout the fibre. Such a fibre can respond to up to 350 impulses per second for short periods without tetany but showing rapid fatigue to 30 per cent of the original tension. The axons supplying impulses to these fibres are large and have a high rate of conduction. They end on 'en plaque' or 'sole plate' single nerve endings.

On the other hand, slow, red tonic fibres produce a sustained contraction when stimulated at rates above 20 impulses per second. They have irregularly arranged fibrils in clumps, owe their red colour to the myoglobin inside the fibre and have plentiful mitochondria. The nerve endings on this type of muscle fibre are multiple, distributed along its length, and described as 'en grappe'. These arise from thinner nerve fibres.

Like skeletal muscle, the EOMs contain muscle spindles and about fifty have been identified near the tendon in a single superior rectus muscle. Nerve impulses along the gamma efferent nerves cause contraction and increase sensitivity to stretch. Stretching stimuli are registered by annulospinal or flower-spray endings and impulses are conveyed up large Group I fibres to the trigeminal ganglion and on up the proximal axon to the reticular formation and the cervical spinal cord.

Suxamethonium and other depolarizing agents

When exposed to acetylcholine, the twitch fibres show a momentary contraction followed by total paralysis associated with depolarization. The tonic fibres, on the contrary, contract in a state of prolonged tetany. Similar responses follow the use of suxamethonium, decamethonium and anticholinesterases such as neostigmine.

The clinical use of suxamethonium causes temporary enophthalmos, a rise in IOP and a fairly central pupil, but with a tendency for divergence and elevation of gaze.

The rise in IOP caused by suxamethonium has been the subject of much investigation. Unfortunately, some of the early work ignored the rise in IOP caused by laryngoscopy and intubation. There was also a lack of understanding of the influence of respiration on IOP. Cook (1981), in a well-controlled investigation on ventilated 'steady-state' patients and using hand-held applanation tonometry, has shown that the pressure rises rapidly during the first minute to about 8 mmHg above the initial level; there is then a gradual fall for five minutes, followed by a final rapid fall to normal within ten minutes of administration. These changes are not dose related for suxamethonium nor are they always blocked by the previous administration of curare as was once thought.

It is interesting to speculate on the causes of the rise in IOP. There is no doubt that increased tension in the tonic fibres of the EOM is part of the mechanism. This was shown as early as 1955 by Lincoff, who observed the inferior oblique contract after the administration of suxamethonium. He also noted 3-mm enophthalmos caused in one patient. His observation that the division of all the EOMs in a dog blocked the rise in IOP is open to the criticism that the ciliary body and the anterior part of the eye obtain most of their blood supply from arteries accompanying the rectus muscles. These vessels enter the eye at the insertion of the muscles into the globe and are vital to the production of aqueous humour and the intraocular circulation.

Suxamethonium causes a slight rise in blood pressure, probably through a nicotinic effect on sympathetic ganglia. It is unlikely that a similar effect makes a major contribution to ocular haemodynamics.

The gradual initial fall in IOP probably results from the drainage of aqueous out of the eye through the trabeculum and this is also suggested by the fact that the rate of fall is similar to that demonstrated in tonography in which a weight is placed on the cornea and the rate of fall is measured.

The second rapid fall corresponds with the hydrolysis of suxamethonium to the much weaker depolarizer succinyl monocholine.

The interesting patient among the forty studied by Cook is one who received only 1 mg/kg, whose pressure remained elevated by 6 mmHg even after 15 minutes. Was there some experimental fault in this case or was there some inherent defect in the patient such as abnormality or deficiency of plasma cholinesterase to delay the breakdown of the suxamethonium? Would this patient have presented problems if an intraocular operation had been attempted?

It has been known for years that prolonged neuromuscular block from suxamethonium may be associated with raised IOP. The causes of such a block include congenital absence of the enzyme plasma cholinesterase, abnormal types of the enzyme, or a deficiency resulting from severe disease or exposure to anticholinesterase drugs or insecticides. The congenital forms of the deficiency have an incidence of 1:3000 patients. The only medically used anticholinesterase drugs likely to be encountered are ecothiopate eyedrops for glaucoma, neostigmine and pyridostigmine. Drugs specifically to prolong the action of suxamethonium, such as tetrahydroamino acrine, have passed into history and are no longer marketed in Britain.

The clinical use of suxamethonium

In spite of the hazards to the eye, the risk of fatal malignant hyperpyrexia, the problems of prolonged apnoea and the severe discomfort of postoperative muscle pain, suxamethonium is still commonly used as the agent to achieve endotracheal intubation before eye surgery. It remains the best relaxant, so far, to provide complete, rapid and temporary relaxation of the jaw and larynx. This facilitates atraumatic intubation in patients with mouths resplendent with the prosthetic art of the dental surgeon, and whose cervical spines have lost their original flexibility.

There are certain precautions that the cautious anaesthetist will take. He will avoid suxamethonium in patients who have evidence of recent exposure to anticholinesterases or who, on investigation, have low plasma cholinesterase. This is not solely for his own benefit, nor simply in the general interest of the patient, but specifically because of the risk of loss of intraocular contents when the eye is opened. It would be wise to restrict the dose of suxamethonium to less than 1 mg/kg. In most cases, with the passage of time, the institution of intermittent positive-pressure ventilation (IPPV) and the administration of halothane or enflurane, IOP falls to a safe level long before the surgeon enters the anterior chamber. In an ideal world, the surgeon would not commence surgery until tonometry had been performed and the exact IOP measured. This is a policy of perfection which is probably not obtainable—however, in the occasional patient, it is an easy and excellent procedure with which the ophthalmic anaesthetist should be familiar. In no circumstances should decamethonium or neostigmine or any other anticholinesterase be used before or during intraocular surgery.

Non-depolarizing relaxants

All non-depolarizing relaxants produce relaxation of the extraocular muscles (EOMs) and permit artificial ventilation of the lungs during intraocular surgery. The differences between different drugs depend on:

speed of onset,
length of action,
autonomic blockade,
histamine release,
ease of reversal.

The oldest standard drug is tubocurarine. It is slow acting, produces ganglionic block and releases histamine locally. Occasionally, dramatic hypotension may occur in elderly patients with the commencement of IPPV when this drug is employed. It should be used in low dosage and with extreme caution when it is suspected that the patient has dysautonomia resulting from age or diabetes.

Pancuronium is relatively free of autonomic or histaminic activity and produces a stable cardiovascular state. Unfortunately, in some elderly patients, particularly those on diuretics, it proves to have a suprisingly long action which is difficult to reverse. Some elderly patients who had received only 6 mg of the drug subsequently required IPPV overnight.

Fazadinium has the advantage of rapid onset but its length of action is rather too great for most simple ophthalmic procedures.

As a personal preference, the author often uses tubocurarine 15 mg and supplements this with halothane, enflurane or fentanyl as necessary. Forty minutes after the initial dose, there is no need to reverse it and this reduces the need for pharyngeal toilet with its attendant coughing, straining and trauma which lead to an uncomfortable recovery. Minimal blind suction with a soft catheter is all that is required, and then not in every case. This contrasts with the practice of the anaesthetist in thoracic or abdominal surgery who, quite usually, performs a thorough pharyngeal toilet on every patient using a laryngoscope. In ophthalmic practice this might be considered meddlesome unless specifically indicated.

References

Cook, J.H. (1981). The effect of suxamethonium on intraocular pressure. *Anaesthesia* **36**, 359.

Davson, H. (1980). *The Physiology of the Eye,* 4th edn. Churchill Livingstone, Edinburgh.

Hess, A. and Pilar, G. (1963). Slow fibres in the extraocular muscles of the cat. *Journal of Physiology* **169**, 780.

Katz, R.L. and Eakins, K.E. (1969). *Proceedings of the Royal Society of Medicine* **62**, 1217.

Last, R.J. (1968). *Eugene Wolff's Anatomy of the Eye and Orbit,* 6th edn. H.K. Lewis, London.

Lincoff, H.A. (1955). The effect of succinylcholine on intraocular pressure. *American Journal of Ophthalmology* **40**, 501.

3

Anaesthesia for cataract surgery

The most common operation in ophthalmic surgery is for the removal of a cataract or opacity of the lens. A mature cataract is shown in Fig. 3.1.

Indications for general anaesthesia

There are still many surgeons who prefer to perform all intraocular operations under local anaesthesia, which is usually administered by the surgeon. It is hardly an exaggeration to say that if the anaesthetist uses a similar delicacy in his techniques of instrumentation as the ophthalmologist, there will seldom be episodes of coughing, straining or vomiting postoperatively, particularly if the patients are carefully prepared and a good anaesthetic technique is pursued.

In Britain, where Von Graefe sections are becoming increasingly uncommon, a surgeon will repair a mechanically sound section under a

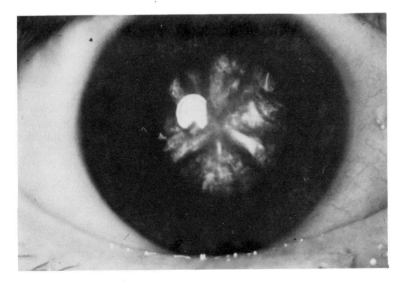

Fig. 3.1 A mature cataract.

microscope with such accurate suturing that mishaps to the eye during or immediately after anaesthesia should be very rare, even if the patient becomes lively in the recovery ward!

The indications for general, as opposed to local, anaesthesia are most powerful when the patient is likely to be uncooperative due to the absence of a common language, deafness, extremes of age, confusion, the pains of arthritis or severe orthopnoea. More relative indications are patient preference, a prolonged surgical technique, medico-legal problems or the training of junior surgeons.

There is no doubt that when the anaesthetic service is good, many more patients are operated on using general anaesthesia; there is no increase in the change-over time between patients; and the operative morbidity and mortality are unchanged, as is shown in a later chapter.

Local anaesthesia

Most anaesthetists working in this field will be familiar with the problem of the patient who appears to be such a poor risk for general anaesthesia that it is suggested that the surgeon should operate under local anaesthesia. The surgeon insists that an operation is only likely to be successful under general anaesthesia and reluctantly the anaesthetist accepts the increased risk. Usually the operation takes place uneventfully. All indications for local anaesthesia are relative and depend on the experience of the anaesthetist and the confidence of the surgeon. Not infrequently, the eye surgeon decides the type of anaesthesia without reference to his anaesthetic colleagues—and occasionally regrets it!

Basal narcosis

The combination of basal narcosis and local anaesthesia has always had its advocates. The techniques are constantly evolving but suffer a number of drawbacks. The airway is unprotected, making the risks of regurgitation and inhalation a constant danger, particularly when the patient has a hiatus hernia. The airway may become partially or completely obstructed beneath the drapes causing snoring, forced respiratory movement or asphyxia.

The level of sedation is difficult to monitor: if the patient is too light, he may be confused or violent; if he is too deep, then there are all the dangers and none of the security of general anaesthesia. Techniques which depend on single doses tend to use long-acting agents which prolong recovery, while infusions tend to produce an uneven level of unconsciousness. Lastly, all these agents tend to produce depression of respiration and a degree of carbon dioxide retention which congests the choroid coat of the eye.

Nevertheless, in some hands, these techniques will remain popular for the older patient despite the obvious dangers and disadvantages. The lytic cocktail of chlorpromazine, promethazine and pethidine was a great advance over previous methods which relied solely on opiates or barbiturates. This technique was replaced in succession by neuroleptanalgesia, intravenous diazepam and infusions of various barbiturates, analgesics and hypnotic steroids. None of these techniques is routinely in use at Moorfields Eye Hospital for cataract surgery at the present time, although variants of these techniques are used occasionally.

The general policy with patients under local anaesthesia is to aim for a relaxed, co-operative patient who has had a small dose of an anxiolytic agent.

The indications for local anaesthesia may be listed as follows:

1. Patient preference (especially when the first eye has been successfully operated on under local anaesthesia).
2. Surgical preference (particularly more senior and faster surgeons).
3. Poor anaesthetic service.
4. Severe systemic disease (common examples are given as illustrations and are not exhaustive).
(a) Neuromuscular disorders: dystrophia myotonica, myasthenia gravis, malignant hyperpyrexia.
(b) Haematological problems: sickle cell disease, thalassaemia minor.
(c) Cardiac decompensation: congestive cardiac failure, recent cardiac infarction.
(d) Respiratory failure: emphysema, chronic bronchitis, pulmonary tuberculosis.
(e) Skeletal deformity: ankylosing spondylitis, fusion of the cervical spine.
(f) Endocrine disorders: diabetes mellitus.
(g) Incompatible medication: monoamine oxidase inhibitors, ecothiopate.
(h) Thromboembolic disorders.
(i) Liver failure: cirrhosis.
(j) Renal failure.

Problems of cataract surgery

The very old

An increasing number of extremely old patients are presenting themselves for cataract surgery. It has, in the past, been argued that the slow progression of senile cataract allows the patient to adapt to his increasing blindness and that such a patient does not always welcome the independence permitted by vision, will not adapt to spherical aberrations caused by the pebble-like aphakic corrections in his spectacles, and would therefore be unlikely to benefit from surgery. The increasing numbers of elderly people who live alone, partly dependent on television and partly on the social activities of a Day Centre, have changed this. The introduction of contact lenses and improved types of intraocular lenses has improved the visual results of surgery. Even in the bedridden and confused patient, operation may lead to improved co-operation and a better quality to the end of life. It is against this background that the balance must be made between an increased quality of living and a fairly small risk of dying. The metabolic disturbance of cataract extraction is very small and the benefits may be considerable.

Confusion

Many elderly patients have been immobilized by blindness for years and, in some of these, there is a degree of preoperative confusion or depression which may be related to loss of vision. Admission to hospital and general anaesthesia may exacerbate this. It is very important that only extremely small doses of central nervous system depressants are given to the elderly. Long-acting agents, in particular, cause problems and the nursing staff may be placed in considerable difficulties when drugs such as hyoscine, promethazine or lorazepam are used in the over-eighties. At this age, many patients are happy with a preoperative visit, reassurance and no premedication.

Prostatism

Patients with symptoms of chronic retention of urine, resulting from enlargement of the prostate gland, are poor candidates for cataract surgery. Eye wards are not ideal places to deal with acute postoperative retention of urine, and it is sound advice for patients with prostatism to have this corrected before having their lens extracted.

Orthostatic oedema

Elderly, blind people tend to sit in a chair for many hours each day. Some of them develop massive oedema of the legs which is quite benign. This orthostatic oedema is frequently confused with congestive cardiac failure, but is distinguished by the lack of other signs or symptoms of cardiac decompensation or renal impairment. Problems do arise when these patients lie horizontal for a few additional hours as they autotransfuse themselves with several litres of extravascular fluid and precipitate acute pulmonary oedema, frequently in the recovery period after anaesthesia. Preoperative prescription of a diuretic for two days before anaesthesia will reduce the risks of pulmonary oedema without completely removing the fluid retained in the legs. This treatment often dramatically improves the postoperative mobility of the patient.

Cardiac disease

Many patients for cataract surgery have a past history of ischaemic heart disease, suffer from angina or are in congestive cardiac failure. There is no doubt that there is an increased risk in such patients whether local or general anaesthesia is employed; but when a correct preoperative assessment has been made, many patients should not be denied surgery or anaesthesia.

Previous cardiac infarction which has not been followed by a permanent disorder of rhythm or cardiac failure carries a good prognosis provided that the danger period of three months, described by Arkins *et al.* (1964), has been allowed to elapse since the cardiac infarction. These patients may well equate with those suffering from ischaemic heart disease whose preoperative clinical assessment was described as 'good' in the survey conducted at Cardiff by Fowkes *et al.* (1982). They recorded a mortality of 1.1 per cent in elective operations for this group, which probably included many major general and orthopaedic procedures. Chronic angina of effort with a stable ECG and normal enzyme tests probably relate to the 'minor impairment' group in the same study and produced a mortality of 1.6 per cent.

Contraindications to elective surgery are angina at rest, increasing frequency of angina, tachycardia with hypertension, raised central venous pressure, depression of serum potassium concentrations, complete heart block, aortic valve incompetence, constrictive pericarditis, and pulmonary hypertension. In such patients, the risk must be carefully weighed by the surgeon, anaesthetist and patient after such remedial measures as are possible have been taken.

Many patients, at about the age of 70, develop an ejection sound on auscultation of the chest which is caused by partial calcification of the aortic valve. The functional activity of such a valve, although reduced, may remain surprisingly good and, in the absence of left ventricular strain or poor left ventricular output, the diagnosis of calcific aortic stenosis should be avoided and surgery should not be withheld.

Cardiac patients should always receive preinduction oxygenation. Oesophageal reflux is common and intubation may be delayed by cervical spondylosis or other factors. Allowance must be made for increased arm–brain circulation time by reducing the speed of injection and all doses, particularly those of induction agents, should be minimal both in terms of absolute dosage and concentration.

Finally, it is important that the anaesthetist shows confidence and that undue anxiety is not conveyed to the patient, who cannot see what is going on and may also be unable to hear.

Dystrophia myotonica

Patients who are unfortunate enough to inherit the sex-linked autosomal dominant gene which produces early cataract, frontal balding, testicular atrophy and muscular dystrophy (sometimes but not always associated with delayed relaxation after voluntary contraction) are a rare but important problem for the ophthalmic anaesthetist. The management of these patients may be summarized as careful preoperative assessment, minimal doses of all depressant agents, particularly thiopentone, avoidance of suxamethonium and reduced doses of non-depolarizing muscle relaxants. It is vital to observe the respiratory function of these patients postoperatively and, if necessary, control ventilation artificially.

Marfan's syndrome

It is well known that patients with this autosomal dominant disorder of connective tissue present to the ophthalmic surgeon with a dislocated lens—sometimes bilaterally. The suspensory ligament becomes progressively weaker and eventually dislocation occurs in nearly all patients with the condition; indeed, it may be the only indication of the disease. However, outside ophthalmic circles it is seldom appreciated that retinal detachment is very frequent and while a dislocated lens may not need an operation, a detachment will always require one to forestall blindness.

The anaesthetist is sometimes faced by a dislocated lens in a very young patient in his teens or twenties. There is not the option of performing an extracapsular extraction of the cataract, and the surgeon must attempt to perform an intracapsular extraction. Not infrequently, the lens slips posteriorly into the vitreous, either spontaneously or as the result of the slightest surgical manoeuvre. Fortunately, the lens usually falls by gravity below the optical axis of the eye and this is equivalent to the archaic operation of 'couching' the cataract. Most surgeons would treat a posteriorly dislocated lens conservatively rather than risk a difficult vitrectomy and extraction. The anaesthetist must use all his skill to keep the vitreous well back in the eye during these procedures, and, even then, a small anterior vitrectomy may be required to close the eye without getting vitreous into the surgical section.

The fully developed case with arachnodactyly and long limbs frequently has a very long neck and even a long-bladed laryngoscope may be barely long enough to reach the larynx. The serious cardio-vascular manifestations of the disease tend to affect the root of the aorta and may cause a dissecting aneurysm or progressive aortic incompetence. Murdock *et al.* (1972) record the average age of death in a series of seventy-two patients as 32 years.

On theoretical grounds, dissection is less likely if fluctuations of blood pressure can be avoided, though in practice the author has been unable to find any reports of dissection following anaesthesia. Aortic incompetence may become rapidly fatal if allowed to become decompensated, and myocardial depressants should not be given rapidly to patients with signs of cardiovascular disease. Pyeritz (1980) recommends the ultrasonic determination of the minimum aortic diameter as a prognostic determination. Values below 40 mm seem to be fairly safe. It is as well to remember that procedures on these patients may be bilateral and multiple.

The anatomy of the lens

The lens is a compound structure consisting of an external capsule suspended by the fibres of the suspensory ligament from the ciliary muscle. Within this capsule is 'soft lens matter' which is strongly hydrophilic. It swells and fluffs up whenever the capsule is opened. In some cataracts this may occur spontaneously to form a tight tumescent bag; this may happen when a cataract is ripe or in cataracts associated with an intraocular foreign body.

Within the soft lens matter lies a hard nucleus which tends to increase in size and density with age.

Cataract extraction

There are two basic operations: firstly, the intracapsular extraction in which the capsule is removed complete with contents, often using a cryoprobe. This operation exposes the vitreous face behind and is difficult and dangerous in young patients, diabetics and myopes as the vitreous face tends to rupture during the cataract extraction leading to vitreous loss and vitreous strands in the incision, in the drainage angle and across the anterior chamber.

The second type of operation is an extracapsular extraction in which the posterior part of the capsule remains. The anterior capsule is incised or excised and the lens matter with the nucleus is irrigated out of the eye. Modern technology has improved this type of operation; the incision can be very small; the nucleus can be broken up by ultrasound; and the lens matter removed by sophisticated methods of irrigation. This is a growth area in ophthalmology and techniques change every year. The risks of vitreous loss are reduced and it seems to be a preferable form of cataract operation prior to the insertion of some types of intraocular lens. In a few patients, the posterior capsule loses transparency and requires incision at a later capsulotomy.

Techniques of anaesthesia

The three aims of a general anaesthetic for cataract extraction can be stated as:

  a quiet and unresponsive patient,
  a quiet and uncongested eye,
  a quiet and rapid recovery.

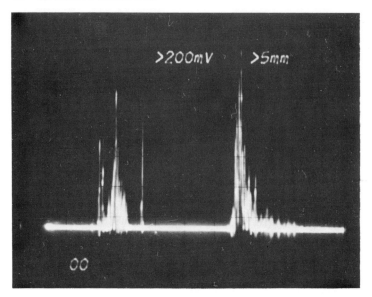

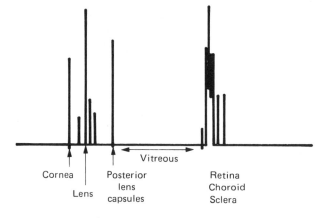

Fig. 3.2 The photographs illustrate the use of ultrasound in the diagnosis of eye disease. They are both 'A' scans. 'A' scans demonstrate the structure of the eye in a single plane. 'B' scans demonstrate stuctures in two planes; and 'M' scans can show changes or movement within the eye. If the posterior coats of the eye are examined in greater detail by

Until a few year ago, the aims were partly achieved by deep anaesthesia. It is now evident that, providing the afferent stimuli are adequately blocked, a light plane of anaesthesia will suffice. Neurosurgical anaesthetists have been aware of the advantages of hyperventilation for much longer than ophthalmic anaesthetists. In the same way that the vascular component of the intracerebal volume can be

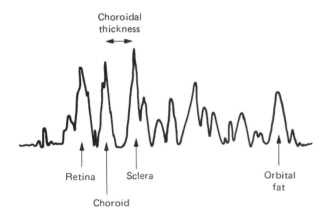

spreading them × 100, the thickness of individual layers may be measured in life and the changes in thickness of the choroid under the influence of alterations in ventilation or the use of drugs may be measured.

shrunk by respiratory alkalosis, so also can the congestion of the erectile tissue of the choroid of the eye be reduced. This can be demonstrated in the elderly patient with good lungs in whom enthusiastic hyperventilation makes the lens lie so far back in the eye that application of the cryoprobe to the lens becomes difficult. A more sophisticated technique is to measure choroidal thickness by ultrasound, as in Fig. 3.2.

Preoperative assessment

There are few absolute contraindications to general anaesthesia—just good risks and poor risks. Aortic sclerosis, angina of effort and ischaemic electrocardiographic traces seem to be universal among the group of patients requiring this type of surgery. With care, gentleness, adequate monitoring and generous oxygenation, these conditions cause few problems.

Remediable conditions such as congestive cardiac failure, myxoedema, chronic bronchitis and anaemia need adequate investigation and preparation before surgery. Failure to diagnose, investigate and treat a medical condition prior to planned surgery renders the anaesthetist open to severe criticism. Should a mishap occur subsequently which might have been avoided if the patient had been brought to the best possible state of health, then allegations of negligence may be made.

There are few routine haematological, biochemical or radiological investigations which need to be done on cataract patients who are symptom free, but no Negro patient should ever be anaesthetized without the investigation of his blood for abnormal haemoglobins. Fortunately, rapid laboratory methods of identifying abnormal haemoglobins are now available to supplement the bedside Sickledex test. The rarity of sickling in patients who are not Negro renders routine screening uneconomic.

Premedication

Drugs used for premedication tend to have a long therapeutic effect and frequently add to the postoperative confusion of a patient who cannot see and sometimes has difficulty in hearing. Hyoscine (Scopolamine) is particularly contraindicated, while promethazine and related drugs need to be used in small doses. Relief of anxiety is a major aim and the use of anxiolytic drugs of the benzodiazepine group is increasing. These are rapidly effective when given orally, and short-acting agents of the series may be an improvement over diazepam and lorazepam.

Although morphine is probably justified in patients who have a smoker's cough, the incidence of nausea and vomiting in susceptible individuals renders its routine use inadvisable, even with an anti-emetic, as the action of the latter is nearly always very short.

A common standard premedication for a 70-year-old patient is frequently promethazine 12.5 mg, pethidine (meperidine) 50 mg and atropine 0.3 mg, one hour before operation In practice, this works well but is pharmacologically open to criticism as promethazine has a half-life of 12 hours, pethidine of 1.5 hours and atropine of 2 hours. The pethidine will hardly help with postoperative analgesia, and sometimes causes preoperative nausea; while the atropine renders the patient's mouth uncomfortably dry.

Those who use oral diazepam find its action too long for a rapid recovery. Intravenous atropine at the time of induction needs to be given in a dose of 1 mg to keep secretions under control.

Induction

There is a wide choice of agents, many of which are suitable. Although etomidate reduces intraocular pressure selectively, as yet there is no firm evidence of its mode of action and no clear advantage in cataract surgery. It may be sensible to avoid drugs known to cause a high incidence of hiccough or spontaneous muscle movement. Barbiturates depress the myocardium and must be given slowly and in low dosage. Alphaxalone-alphadone is a useful agent, but hypersensitivity causing bronchospasm and hypotension may occur. It is best reserved as an alternative agent rather than the drug of first choice.

Intubation

The choice of muscle relaxant for this procedure is becoming increasingly controversial as suxamethonium may, rarely, trigger malignant hyperpyrexia or cause prolonged apnoea because the patient has a congenital or acquired deficiency of serum cholinesterase. It frequently causes back and chest pain postoperatively. Intubation following its use is invariably easier than it is with other relaxants owing to the rapid onset of almost total muscular paralysis. Its usual short duration of action allows spontaneous respiration to take place during surgery.

The rise in IOP following its use does not last more than six minutes from the time of injection and is probably not significant unless plasma cholinesterase levels are abnormally low (in which case the IOP stays elevated for a longer period). It has been argued that the return of IOP to normal after suxamethonium is dependent on drainage of aqueous from the eye and the factors causing the initial rise in pressure, such as tetanus of the extraocular muscles, may last much longer than the rise in IOP.

Becaue of these disadvantages, there is something to be gained in using a non-depolarizing relaxant of rapid onset such as fazadinium. This would not be appropriate if spontaneous respiration was required, owing to its length of action.

Endotracheal intubation

Ideally, this should be rapid and atraumatic. Many anaesthetists still spray the vocal cords with lignocaine 4%, well knowing that the local anaesthetic action will have passed off before extubation takes place, arguing that the patients settle more easily under anaesthesia and that the transient rise in IOP on intubation is reduced by surface anaesthesia. The lubrication of the tube with local anaesthetic gel or water-miscible cream

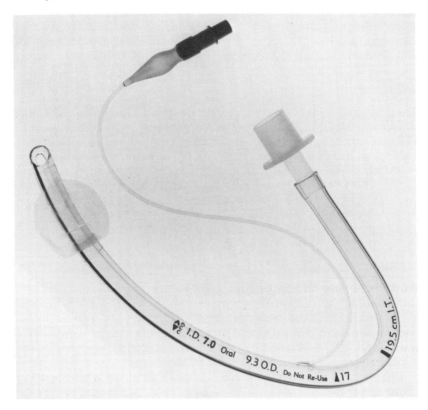

Fig. 3.3 A RAE endotracheal tube produced by Mallinckrodt. These are much less inclined to kink than Magill tubes.

seems to be just as effective.

The tube itself is liable to kink and obstruct on the posterior surface of the tongue and there is a strong argument for using a latex tube reinforced with a nylon or metal helix. Very good preformed RAE tubes of disposable plastic are produced by Mallinckrodt (Fig. 3.3); they are rather expensive for single use. An alternative would be to use one of the many varieties of armoured or reinforced tubes available on the market, such as the very long tube shown in Fig. 3.4.

Positioning of the table

The patient for cataract extraction lies supine with his head supported in the depression of a Ruben's pillow. This pillow forms a flat surface

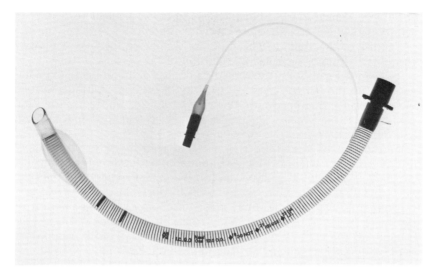

Fig. 3.4 An armoured tube. This tube is long enough to come down over the chin. However, it requires very accurate positioning to avoid intubation of the right bronchus.

under the towels to provide a rest for the surgeon's forearms and for the instruments actually in use. Its main defect is that it moves considerably under pressure as it rests on the table mattress.

There are ventilatory advantages to tipping up the head of the table about five degrees. It relieves the pressure of abdominal contents on the diaphragm; it is a valuable means of decongesting the eye; and, in very fat patients, a steeper tilt may be beneficial. It is a good aphorism that 'the eye should be above the heart'. In other words, venous pressure in the orbit should be atmospheric.

Maintenance

The choice between spontaneous or artificial ventilation is important. Almost all cataracts are more safely removed with IPPV to lower the arterial carbon dioxide tension. The younger the patient, the more important this becomes. Unfortunately, in a number of patients, the rapid introduction of the Valsalva effect of IPPV with large tidal volumes immediately after a barbiturate induction (particularly with tubocurarine and halothane) leads to a frightening depression of the blood pressure. This effect is partly due to the dysautonomia in the patient caused by old age or diabetic neuropathy, partly to the ganglionic-blocking and histamine-releasing action of tubocurarine and partly to the cardiodepressant action of the induction agent followed by halothane. This can be prevented by the use of great care and low doses or by using other sequences such as droperidol, pancuronium and enflurane. Pancuronium sometimes seems to be difficult to reverse in elderly patients, especially those receiving diuretics.

The use of this type of technique has eliminated the risk of massive choroidal haemorrhage causing expulsion of the ocular contents.

To achieve a satisfactory carbon dioxide level of about Paco$_2$ 4kPa it is very useful, though not essential, to monitor the end-expiratory carbon dioxide using a capnograph. Raised levels are an indication that ventilation is inadequate. The cause should be sought so that vitreous loss during cataract surgery may be avoided.

At the end of operation, it is wise to restrict the inspection and aspiration of the pharynx to a minimum in order to prevent heaving and coughing. Although in anaesthesia for abdominal surgery it is the rule, automatically, to reverse curare with neostigmine, in eye surgery profound muscle relaxation may not be necessary in the last minute of the operation. It is possible, on many occasions, to so time and adjust the dosage of muscle relaxant and to supplement it with respiratory depressants such as fentanyl or halothane that there is no need to reverse the relaxant given 40 minutes earlier. This avoids neostigmine-induced secretions.

Spontaneous respiration is best reserved for patients over 70 or those who have pulmonary cavities or bullae. The older patient has a shrunken vitreous and a rigid sclera which render vitreous loss unlikely in the absence of coughing or straining.

Postoperative care

Cataract patients used to be nursed supine with their head supported between sandbags for several days postoperatively. This is no longer the case and most patients are mobilized under supervision on the same day as the operation. Some surgeons do leave a bubble of air in the anterior chamber of the eye and these patients should be nursed supine for fear that air may pass through the pupil and lodge behind the iris, which it will balloon forward so as to block the drainage of aqueous through the angle. With this exception, there is no objection to patients being put into the 'safe' or lateral position, preferably with the operated eye uppermost. Cataract extraction does not cause severe pain postoperatively and only about 30 per cent of patients require analgesics. A similar proportion receive an anti-emetic on request, but not routinely.

Osmotic agents and acetazolamide

There is a declining use of osmotic agents in cataract surgery. Various centres have tried the effects of urea, sucrose and mannitol, particularly on young patients in whom difficulties were expected. The surgeon was seldom disappointed and difficulties were often encountered!

There is some experimental evidence that osmotic agents reduce the size of the vitreous body in baboons. This reduction is small because the vitreous is avascular and osmotic agents have more influence on highly vascular organs, such as the brain or cells in the blood, for example erythrocytes. The water drawn out of the cells in the more vascular parts of the body increases the volume of the extravascular fluid compartment by up to 80 per cent of the original value and much of this is taken up by an increase in the circulating blood volume. The rise in central venous pressure and the vasodilatation of the choroid more than compensate for the shrinkage of the vitreous. To make matters worse, the operative field is rendered more vascular than usual.

Acetazolamide has been used on the grounds that it reduces IOP and this must be good. It acts solely by reducing the secretion of aqueous humour and has no influence on the vitreous. It has been shown by Wilson et al. (1977) that this drug increases choroidal blood flow by two or three times the normal value for about 50 minutes; as a result, it more than negates any advantage.

Keratoplasty

Corneal grafting, or keratoplasty, presents all the problems of cataract surgery but these are magnified. In this operation, a full-thickness disc is excised from the cornea and replaced by a donor disc of the same size which has usually been cut from a cadaver within a short time of death. The disc is accurately sewn in place and the end-results of such a procedure can be seen in Fig. 3.5.

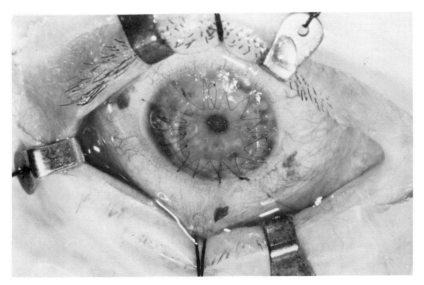

Fig. 3.5 A corneal graft. The elasticity of the nylon suture and the accuracy of the suturing allow the patient to get out of bed within a few hours of operation.

For the anaesthetist, the problem is to provide an eye initially which is hard enough to be cut with the trephine, but once the disc has been cut the eye is totally unprotected against any change in orbital or intraocular pressure such as might be provoked by coughing, straining or breathing against the ventilator. There is at this stage a major risk of loss of intraocular contents. The patient must be totally relaxed and all reflexes depressed until the stitching has been completed, the tension in the suture adjusted and the last knot tied. A few of the patients who require this operation were blinded by mustard gas in the Great War and have extensive residual lung damage which makes the control of cough during anaesthesia very difficult.

References

Arkins, R., Smessaert, A.A. and Hicks, R.G. (1964). Mortality and morbidity in surgical patients with coronary artery disease. *Journal of the American Medical Association* **190**, 485.

Bettman, J.W. and Fellows, V.G. (1956). Factors influencing the blood volume of the choroid and retina. *Transactions of the American Academy of Ophthalmology and Otolaryngology* **60**, 791,

Blackburn, C.L. and Morgan, M. (1978). Comparison of speed of onset of fazadinium, pancurorium, tubocurarine and suxamethonium. *British Journal of Anaesthesia* **50**, 361.

Coleman, D.J. and Lizzi, F. (1979). In vivo choroidal thickness measurement. *American Journal of Ophthalmology* **88**, 369.

Cook, J.H. (1981). The effect of suxamethonium on intraocular pressure. *Anaesthesia* **36**, 359.

Fowkes, F.G.R., Lunn, J.N., Farrow, S.C., Robertson, I.B. and Samuel, P. (1982). Mortality risk in patients with coexisting physical disease. *British Journal of Anaesthesia* **54**, 819.

Holloway, K.B. (1980). The anaesthetist and the control of intraocular pressure. *British Journal of Anaesthesia* **52**, 671.

MacDiarmid, I.R. and Holloway, K.B. (1976). Factors affecting intraocular pressure. *Proceedings of the Royal Society of Medicine* **69**, 601.

Murdoch, J.L., Walker, B.A., Halpern, B.L., Zuyma, J.W. and McKusick, V.A. (1972). Life expectancy and causes of death in the Marfan Syndrome. *New England Journal of Medicine* **286**, 804.

Oji, E.O. and Holdcroft, E. (1979). The ocular effects of etomidate. *Anaesthesia* **34**, 245.

Pandey, K., Badola, R.P. and Kumar, S. (1972). Time course of intraocular hypertension produced by suxamethonium. *British Journal of Anaesthesia* **44**, 191.

Pyeritz, R.E. (1980). Diagnosis and management of cardiovascular disorders in the Marfan Syndrome. *Journal of Cardiovascular Medicine* **5**, 759.

Samuel, J.R. and Beaugie, A. (1974). Effect of carbon dioxide on the intraocular pressure in man during general anaesthesia. *British Journal of Ophthalmology* **58**, 62.

Smith, R.B., Auss, A.A. and Nemeto, E.M. (1981). Intraocular and intracranial pressure during respiratory ankalosis and acidosis. *British Journal of Anaesthesia* **55**, 967.

Taylor, T.H., Mulcahy, M. and Nightingale, D. (1968). Suxamethonium chloride in intraocular surgery. *British Journal of Anaesthesia* **40**, 113.

Wilson, T.M., Strong, R. and MacKenzie, E.T. (1977). The response of the choroidal and cerebral circulations to changing arterial P_{CO_2} and acetazolamide in the baboon. *Investigations of Ophthalmology and Visual Sciences* **16**, 576.

4

Diabetes and vitrectomy

Diabetes in an eye hospital

Diabetics form about 30 per cent of all ophthalmic in-patients but only a third of these are insulin dependent, the remainder being controlled by a combination of diet and oral hypoglycaemic agents. Many eye units are small in size and often geographically isolated from a general hospital; this renders the management of the disease difficult and sometimes dangerous. Quite large ophthalmic hospitals lack the basic facilities of a dietician and a diet kitchen; an endocrinologist may attend one or two days a week but the continuity of care is placed on the shoulders of the ophthalmic surgeon, his junior staff and, immediately preceding and following the operation, the anaesthetist.

The problem has been thrown into prominence during the last three years, since many diabetics, previously considered inoperable by the surgeons, are now admitted for surgery. Apart from their eye condition they often suffer from varying degrees of renal failure, vascular problems, neuropathy and not infrequently have lost one or both lower limbs. There is much to be said in favour of grouping the insulin-dependent patients in the same area of the hospital or even, as advocated recently by Walts *et al.* (1981), of setting up a diabetic intensive care unit. This would only be practical in a very large eye hospital.

In order to concentrate medical and nursing resources on the patients most in need of skilled care, it is necessary to perform a triage or sorting procedure on diabetic patients.

Firstly, the patients controlled solely by diet present no problem provided their diet is rigidly controlled in hospital and that they do not suffer from some infection which may disturb the balance of their metabolism. Simple starvation before operation and any suitable conventional anaesthetic technique will see these patients safely through the operative period.

The management of patients treated with tablets

The second group, on oral hypoglycaemic agents, seldom presents major problems providing, once again, the diet is controlled. Unfortunately it is true that some patients on tablets would be better controlled by insulin and it is sometimes better to transfer to insulin therapy for the length of the stay in hospital. Some of the oral agents present special problems for the anaesthetist. There are still a few patients whose diabetes is controlled using phenformin. This drug is potentially dangerous when associated with anaesthesia as the lethal complication of lactic acidosis may be provoked, up to several days postoperatively. It should be replaced by a safer drug, several days before surgery. The hypoglycaemic drugs have differing lengths of action and may be potentiated by the concomitant administration of other drugs such as acetazolamide, sulphonamides or beta-blockers. It is safe to continue oral treatment providing the following safety procedures are observed.

1. No oral agent should be given in the 12-hour period before operation.
2. The blood sugar should always be measured one hour before operation. If this is less than 5 mmol/litre, then the operation should be delayed until intravenous glucose has been used to produce a higher figure.
3. All patients with a low blood sugar should receive an infusion of 5% dextrose until a more satisfactory level of blood sugar has been established for some hours.
4. Oral therapy is seldom necessary until the first postoperative meal has been taken.

The drug most commonly associated with long periods of hypoglycaemia is chlorpropamide, but this seldom causes trouble if the safety regime is followed.

Some patients on tablets seem to show a brisk hyperglycaemic response following their admission to hospital and preparation for surgery. There seems to be a psychological triggering mechanism for this, mediated through anxiety promoting the endogenous secretion of adrenaline. The use of anxiolytic agents may reduce the reaction but the anaesthetist is often left with the decision of whether to embark on insulin therapy during the operative period. Fortunately, as ketones are seldom produced by these patients, they are not in serious danger. A personal policy is to resort to a highly purified insulin if the blood sugar exceeds 10 mmol/litre. Ten units are given every hour with a 5% glucose infusion until the blood sugar has stabilized between 6 mmol/litre and 8 mmol/litre. The patient can usually return to oral therapy once the immediate operative period has passed.

Management of diabetics dependent on insulin

Before admission
Diabetics frequently become unstable in the environment of hospital, requiring more insulin; and, providing the management of the disease at

recurrent vitreous haemorrhages, particulartly in homozygote sickle cell disease, HbSS, and in the combination, HbSC.

Local anaesthesia should always be considered; even in the relatively benign heterozygous sickle cell trait, HbAS, Dalal *et al.* (1974), report that a Black male aged 12 years developed aphasia and right hemiplegia shortly after bilateral cryotherapy for retinal lattice degeneration. When general anaesthesia is essential, even in trait, the most experienced anaesthetist available should be obtained; preoxygenation for at least five minutes should take place before induction; the airway and ventilation should not be compromised; and a high inspired oxygen tension maintained. Postoperatively, oxygen therapy should continue for 30 minutes.

Sickle cell disease, HbSS or HbSC, is potentially and unpredictably lethal with or without anaesthesia. Unfortunately, local anaesthetics have too short an action for vitrectomy operations, particularly as adrenaline or other local vasoconstrictors are contraindicated. General anaesthesia may be made safer by performing a partial exchange transfusion using a cell exchange technique three days before operation. The object is to obtain a normal haemoglobin level with at least 50 per cent HbA. There is little evidence that infusions of bicarbonate improve the prognosis and low-molecular-weight dextrans only improve local perfusion.

Vitrectomy

Description of the vitreous humour

The normal vitreous humour has a consistency resembling raw white of egg. In the normal eye, it is situated in the posterior chamber. It tends to have areas where it becomes dense and other areas where it is fluid. When diseased or injured, it may undergo change to fibrous tissue which forms bands inside the eye. These can exert traction on the retina or distort the iris. It may become opaque with membranes formed of scar tissue or contain the results of recent or old haemorrhage arising from the retina or choroid. It sometimes bulges forward after the extraction of a cataract to block the pupil; it may interfere in the healing of a wound and occasionally provides an antigenic source for the autoimmune reaction called sympathetic ophthalmia.

'Open sky' vitrectomy

After a cataract extraction, the vitreous may bulge forward and enter the surgical wound. This is most likely to occur in myopic patients. As vitreous impairs the healing of the section, the surgeon must perform an adequate toilet of the wound edges by drawing vitreous up on to a swab and then excising the strands of vitreous which are left adhering to the swab. This process can be carried out repeatedly through the pupil to any desired extent, but tends to be a rather crude and blind procedure limited to the anterior part of the posterior chamber.

Recent technology has refined the process by introducing motorized suction cutters, or 'vitreous gobblers', which enable more accurate excision of vitreous to take place without pulling on the retina. This procedure only requires a similar anaesthetic to that needed for cataract extraction.

Closed vitrectomy

The most sophisticated techniques are those performed through a series of sclerotomies in the pars plana—that is, the area behind the ciliary body but anterior to the attachment of the retina. Through these openings it is possible to maintain the IOP by an infusion at constant pressure; microsurgical cutters, scissors, ultrasonic fragmenters, suckers and diathermy can be introduced by direct vision into the eye so that accurate dissection can take place. It is common to use a fibreoptic light source in the eye and a contact lens is used on the cornea to improve the definition through the operating microscope.

Anaesthetic problems

Many of the patients are old, sick and diabetic but others have received trauma to the eye. The operations last many hours and a non-toxic anaesthetic technique must be used which is safe in near darkness. The head must be held rigidly so that no movement takes place and the airway must be impeccable. Because of the length of the procedure, great care must be taken of the pressure areas and the subcutaneous nerves (such as the ulnar and the lateral popliteal) which are liable to pressure injury.

The anaesthetist finds that access to the patient is restricted by the amount of apparatus utilized by the surgeon and it is very important that adequate preparations are made during the induction period to place all monitoring apparatus, probes and intravenous lines before the operation starts.

Controlled ventilation with nitrous oxide supplemented by non-depolarizing relaxants and synthetic narcotics seems to be the most effective technique. The airway is best protected by a preformed endotracheal tube with a low-pressure cuff to avoid the danger of pressure necrosis on the tracheal mucosa. The head is strapped to a hard head support and movement is prevented by adjustable rests. The non-operated eye is protected by closing the lids and sometimes the application of a pad. Ideally, the patient's body lies on a foam mattress 8 cm thick, such as is used in neurosurgery. The arms and legs have pressure points carefully padded and the calves of the legs are suspended freely by raising the heels on foam pads. The usual ECG monitor, blood-pressure cuff and intravenous lines are established. Hourly measurements of blood sugar are made on diabetic patients.

During the course of the procedure, vitreous is usually replaced by a saline solution; but when it is necessary to replace a detached retina, it is sometimes necessary to replace vitreous with air, sulphur hexafluoride gas or silicone oil.

It is important to emphasize the danger of using nitrous oxide anaesthesia whenever vitreous is replaced by air or sulphur hexafluoride gas (Stinson *et al.* 1982). Since nitrous oxide is extremely soluble, it will diffuse rapidly into a body space containing a less soluble gas—thus causing rapid expansion of the gas-filled space. Smith *et al.* (1974) reported a rise of IOP from 17 mmHg to 39 mmHg in a rhesus monkey who had had 0.5 ml of vitreous replaced by air and was then ventilated with 75% nitrous oxide. It is quite common to inject larger volumes (such as 4 ml) into human eyes. The resulting rise in pressure may cause ischaemia of the retina. This was vividly reported by Fuller and Lewis (1975) who had injected 2.25 ml of 40% sulphur hexafluoride in air during the first operation. The patient was re-anaesthetized with nitrous oxide for an hour to permit a further procedure when they, fortunately, noticed the hardness of the eye and the pallor of the optic disc in time to preserve the vision in the eye by performing a decompression. There may be rare occasions when a non-ophthalmic condition necessitates surgery under general anaesthesia soon after an eye operation. When air or gas remains in the eye, nitrous oxide should be avoided. Similar hazards are involved in air transport of a patient as the pressurization systems of aircraft are usually arranged to mimic atmospheric pressure at 2000 m above sea level.

Administrative problems

The length of this type of operation has a major influence on the pattern of working of an ophthalmic operating theatre as each vitrectomy may replace several shorter operations. This change, in turn, has its own influence on bed occupancy and waiting lists.

The anaesthetist has particular problems as he usually lacks facilities to monitor the progress of the operation or to estimate the length of the procedure. Access to the patient, the airway, the infusion site and the monitoring probes is very limited. For the major part of the operation, the theatre is blacked out or the lighting reduced. The problems of fatigue, boredom and inattention cannot be ignored, neither can those of motivation and recruitment of suitable anaesthetists for this important but tedious work.

References

Dalal, F.Y., Schmidt, G.B., Bennett, E.J. and Ramamurthy, S. (1974). *British Journal of Anaesthesia* **46**, 387.
Fuller, D. and Lewis, M.L. (1975). Nitrous oxide anaesthesia with gas in the vitreous cavity. *American Journal of Ophthalmology* **80**, 778.
Smith, R.B., Carl, B.S., Linn, J.G. and Nemoto, E. (1974). Effect of nitrous oxide on air in vitreous. *American Journal of Ophthalmology* **78**, 315.
Stinson, T.W. and Donlon, J.V. (1982). Interaction of intraocular air and sulfur hexafluoride with nitrous oxide: a computer simulation. *Anesthesiology* **56**, 385.

5

Anaesthetic management of perforating injury

The nature of the injury

The globe of the eye may be penetrated by sharp objects such as sticks, darts, glass fragments or fishhooks. This type of injury tends to cause a cleanly incised laceration of the cornea which becomes plugged with a herniation of iris. A small laceration of this nature may be fairly symptomless and if the iris plug is complete, anaesthetic procedures seldom cause loss of intraocular contents. With very large lacerations the aqueous humour, lens and vitreous may all have been lost before surgery.

The eye may have been bombarded by high-velocity fragments from chiselling, drilling and grinding operations, with multiple fragments from explosions or by gunshot. It is always surprising that a tiny fragment of steel from a chisel can achieve sufficient velocity to penetrate cornea, lens and eventually embed itself in the retina—however, this is one of the commonest indications for emergency surgery on the eye. The entry wound may be so small as to be undetectable. These patients will require radiology or ultrasound or computerized tomography before surgery to localize foreign bodies.

The operations may be prolonged and complicated. In the case of steel foreign bodies, very powerful magnets are employed. The anaesthetist is recommended to use plastic or brass endotracheal tube connecters and to avoid the use of artery forceps or towel clips near the head of the patient. Oscilloscopes, wrist watches and other equipment likely to be damaged in strong magnetic fields should be kept at least 2 m from the operative site.

The third cause of perforating injury is by blunt force. Such trauma is associated with gross haemorrhage and retinal oedema within the globe as well as 'blow-out' fractures of the orbit into the ethmoid sinuses or the maxillary antrum. Such complicated injuries are usually treated in stages; firstly, to restore the integrity of the globe; secondly, to remove blood-stained vitreous; and lastly to repair the orbital walls.

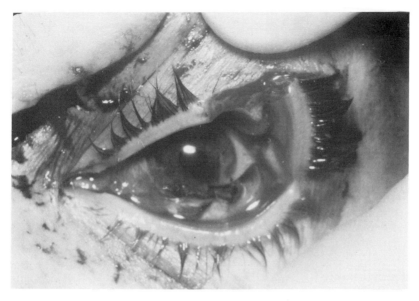

Fig. 5.1 This corneal laceration shows a typical appearance with prolapse of the iris and 'peaking' of the pupil.

Timing of operation

The surgeon will usually be anxious to operate within 12 hours of injury or sooner, to assess the damage, remove foreign bodies and restore the integrity of the globe. This will reduce the risks of infection and also sympathetic ophthalmia which is an autoimmune response to ocular contents which causes an inflammatory uveitis which affects both eyes and may lead to blindness.

The anaesthetist is faced with the general problems of emergency anaesthesia for a recent accident which may include:

1. recent head injury and cerebral oedema;
2. associated injury to the facial skeleton, cervical spine or teeth;
3. injuries to the chest wall, abdomen and limbs (particularly blast lung in the injuries from explosions);
4. hypovolaemic shock from overt or concealed blood loss;
5. nervous shock with sympathetic overactivity;
6. full stomach with inhibition of digestion and ingested blood;
7. alcohol or drug overdose.

The anaesthetist usually has more recent experience of such problems than the eye surgeon and should give appropriate advice and seek help from relevant specialists.

Anaesthetic problems

The anaesthetist must aim to prevent further loss of intraocular contents and provide the surgeon with optimal conditions in which to effect his examination and repair. Every case must be treated seriously and even apparently trivial lacerations need proper anaesthesia with endotracheal intubation.

Ocular contents may be lost as the result of:

1. pressure from an ill-fitting face mask;
2. blepharospasm;
3. orbital pressure from coughing, straining, struggling, airway obstruction, bad posture and obesity;
4. spasm of the extraocular muscles in very light anaesthesia or induced by suxamethonium or decamethonium;
5. choroidal congestion from raised CO_2, anoxia, acetazolamide or intubation.

Management

A careful preoperative assessment must include the taking of a history, a complete examination of the entire patient (except the eye which the surgeon will have already superficially examined using some local anaesthetic instilled into the conjunctival sac) and any necessary special investigations.

Premedication should be given parenterally; absorption from the gastrointestinal tract being unreliable in these patients. Metoclopramide 5 mg may be useful as it doubles the tension in the cardiac sphincter while assisting gastric emptying through the pylorus. It is doubtful whether an antacid or cimetidine is ever really indicated to prevent aspiration pneumonitis in ophthalmic patients as it is usually possible to fast the patient for four to six hours preoperatively.

There is a good case for giving glycopyrrolate or atropine in the premedication, partly to reduce secretions, partly to inhibit the oculocardiac reflex and partly to reduce gastric acidity.

Induction

The safe induction of anaesthesia must be safe for the whole patient as well as preventing further loss of the contents of the globe. The casualty should be treated as a patient potentially at risk from aspiration of gastric contents. An intravenous needle may be inserted during a generous period of preoxygenation. Preoxygenation is very important as it is almost impossible to inflate the patient's lungs using a face mask without exerting pressure on the injured eye.

The eye is placed in jeopardy by techniques utilizing a steep head-down tilt or intubation in the lateral position and even more so if strenuous efforts are made to empty the stomach by using emetics or a gastric tube. The slightly increased risk of regurgitation must be balanced against the ease and speed with which intubation can usually by performed in the supine, horizontal position; confidence being placed in firm continuous cricoid pressure applied by an assistant.

Induction agents generally reduce intraocular tension and there is little to choose between them. Because neuroleptic agents tend to maintain the tone in facial muscles, it may be best not to use these for induction. Ketamine is definitely contraindicated. Thiopentone remains a standard against which other agents can be judged. There are some theoretical advantages in the use of etomidate which lowers intraocular pressure more effectively than thiopentone.

A recent paper by Van Aken et al. (1982) compared topical local anaesthesia of the larynx with the administration of intravenous lignocaine in preventing the rise of intracranial pressure caused by laryngoscopy and intubation. This may well be relevant in anaesthesia for perforating eye injuries and, if confirmed, the induction agent may be followed by lignocaine 1.5 mg/kg. Other methods of achieving the same objective include pretreatment with a small dose of fentanyl as suggested by Kautto (1982).

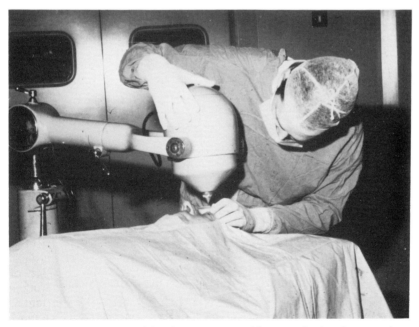

Fig. 5.2 The size and weight of the electromagnet used for extracting iron fragments from the eye make manoeuvrability difficult.

   Suxamethonium and decamethonium are not suitable muscle relaxants if there is an appreciable communication between the inside and outside of the globe. When there has been penetration by only a small spicule of metal, little harm is likely to ensue. Fig. 5.2 shows an electromagnet used to manipulate fragments of iron or steel within the eye to facilitate their removal.

   There do not seem to be absolute differences between the numerous curare-like agents currently available and, as new drugs are constantly being marketed, it is sufficient to remark that the ideal agent should produce profound neuromuscular blockade very rapidly, be free of side-effects on the heart and blood vessels, and be capable of complete and rapid reversal.

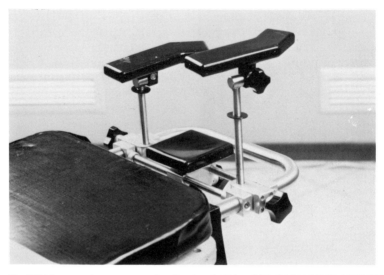

Fig. 5.3 Microscopic surgery needs a firm headrest in which the head is clamped. This rest, designed by Mr Arthur Steele for corneal surgery, is even better for vitrectomy. The anaesthetist has no access to the airway once the patient is towelled up.

   From the moment of induction until intubation is complete, a competent assistant should apply cricoid pressure, and pharyngeal suction should be working and instantly available.

   The repair is usually performed by the surgeon using an operating microscope. To minimize movement of the patient's head a rigid headrest such as that illustrated in Fig. 5.3 is very valuable for the surgeon but even further restricts access for the anaesthetist. This headrest, originally designed for corneal grafting, is suitable for all microscopic surgery.

Maintenance

On general principles, it is convenient to continue anaesthesia with non-depolarizing relaxants, narcotics, nitrous oxide and small amounts of a volatile agent. Hyperventilation should keep the operating conditions good. The blood pressure should be restrained by varying the concentration of inhaled halothane, ethrane or isoflurane. The blood pressure should be maintained at 10–20 mmHg less than the preoperative value so that fresh haemorrhage is not provoked in the eye. Nitrous oxide may have to be discontinued if air or gas is injected to replace lost contents of the eye. The difficulties of access for the anaesthetist are demonstrated in Fig. 5.4 which shows a post-traumatic victrectomy in progress.

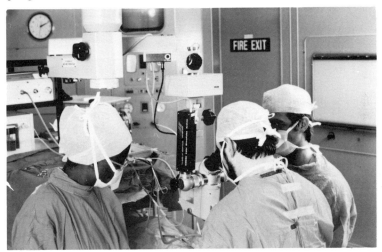

Fig. 5.4 A vitrectomy in progress. There is no access for the anaesthetist. The operating theatre is usually in darkness.

Postoperatively, no special regime can be recommended for this diverse group of patients. A proportion return to the operating theatre within a short period to have the injured eye enucleated, to have a cataractous lens removed, or for treatment of a retinal detachment. It is obviously vital that accurate records from the first anaesthetic are available for subsequent procedures and that they contain all the relevant information.

References

Kautto, U.M. (1982). Attenuation of the circulating response to laryngoscopy and intubation by fentanyl. *Acta anaesthesiologica Scand.*, **26**, 21.

Van Aken, H., Puchstein, C. and Hidding, J. (1982). The prevention of hypertension at intubation. *Anaesthesia*, **37**, 82.

6

Anaesthesia for lacrimal and orbital surgery

Lacrimal surgery

Surgical interventions on the lacrimal drainage system, situated in the medial wall of the orbit, incorporate all the technical difficulties of performing delicate and precise surgical manoeuvres in a highly vascular area through a small surgical exposure while, at the same time, providing the added hazards of ENT surgery such as inhalation of blood, debris and infected material.

Among the patients presenting themselves for this type of surgery are three main groups. The first comprises a number of babies and small children with facial abnormalities, non-patency of the nasolacrimal duct, congenital absence of part of the system or sometimes mongol children. This group occasionally provides the anaesthetist with difficult problems with intubation or associated with abnormalities in other systems such as congenital heart disease.

The second group is made up of young adults who usually require this type of surgery as the result of trauma, particularly windscreen injuries from road traffic accidents. The enthusiastic lacrimal surgeon may wish to perform an emergency repair of a torn canaliculus on a patient who has recently sustained a major head injury. It is important for the anaesthetist to approach such patients with great caution in view of the possibility of a full stomach and intracranial problems such as cerebral oedema, apart from the usual difficulties of associated injury to the neck, thorax or abdomen. A period of delay before surgery is frequently justified to allow surgery to take place under optimal conditions.

Lastly, very elderly patients sometimes require lacrimal drainage to eradicate persistent infection of the sac so that infected material cannot accidentally regurgitate during cataract extraction. To the occasional ophthalmic anaesthetist, lacrimal operations appear to have a low priority and the risks of a fairly lengthy procedure in a frail patient with multiple pathology may seem to be hardly justified. However, a constantly watering eye and recurrent abscess formation in the lacrimal sac produce considerable misery for these patients and there is no satisfactory alternative to surgery. The operation of dacrocysto-rhinostomy (DCR) carried out on a patient with an obstructed nasolacrimal duct has a success rate in excess of 90 per cent and leaves a very grateful patient. Anaesthetists are therefore under some pressure from both patient and surgeon to face the burden of providing anaesthesia, albeit reluctantly, for patients who would appear to be otherwise unfit.

Lacrimal probing and syringing

This seemingly quick simple procedure, performed on a baby, has the ingredients for anaesthetic tragedy. The nasolacrimal duct is often obstructed by a thin membrane near the point of entry into the nose. The lacrimal sac is distended to several times its normal size by mucopus, and mucoceles may form as diverticuli from the sac. When the surgeon's probe has pierced the obstruction and the contents of the sac have been expressed or irrigated through into the nose, the pus may rush into the nasopharynx and be inhaled. The author has seen one non-intubated baby whose bronchi were so choked by secretion that a cardiac arrest occured when the child was turned on its side at the conclusion of the procedure. Another baby inhaled mucus round an endotracheal tube that was too small and developed acute respiratory embarrassment.

The golden rule is always to take these procedures seriously and accordingly never to delegate them to a tyro anaesthetist. Children must always have the airway protected by an endotracheal tube of adequate size and, as an added precaution, the child should be postured so that the pharynx is lower than the trachea as in a tonsillectomy.

Perhaps posture is the most important factor and may suffice in some patients by itself, particularly when the size of the mucocele is small and when some reflexes are preserved such as when ketamine 4–5 mg/kg intramuscularly (i.m.) is employed instead of the more traditional ether or halothane.

As previously noted, some of these children have associated deformity of the face and other defects such as atrial septal defects of the heart. There is a theoretical risk of bacteraemia during probing, and endocarditis could probably occur at a later date.

The lacrimal puncta of babies are frequently hard to locate and may be absent. The surgeon may routinely use a microscope or may need to set one up during the procedure, thus extending the operating time.

In summary, it is highly desirable to use a formal endotracheal anaesthetic and to use an absorbent pharyngeal pack and posture to protect the airway. This provides good surgical access, extended operating time and the ability to use scavenging systems for exhaled vapours. A meticulous pharyngeal toilet should conclude the procedure.

Dacrocystogram (DCG)

The outlining of the lacrimal system by contrast medium enables the surgeon to identify the point of obstruction. (The dacrocystogram in

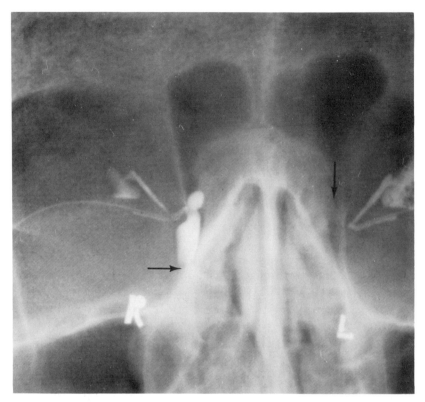

Fig. 6.1 A dacryocystogram (DCG) demonstrating a block of the common canaliculus on the left and the nasolacrimal duct on the right.

Fig. 6.1 shows a block at different sites on the left and right sides.) In children, this can be done under general anaesthesia with all the precautions taken for a probing. The head must remain still and the airway should be protected during the taking of x-rays. Because there is a block, it is unusual for contrast to enter the nose on the obstructed side. If the system is unobstructed, the volume of dye injected, 2 ml, is not significant from a respiratory point of view. The principal hazards are those of hypersensitivity to the contrast medium, respiratory obstruction, and interruption of the oxygen supply while the anaesthetist is sheltering from the radiation.

Dacryocystorhinostomy (DCR)

The operation creates an anastomosis between the lacrimal sac through a surgical fenestration of the nasal bone into the nose and is shown

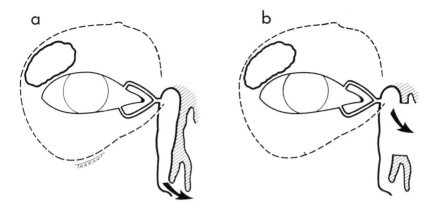

Fig. 6.2 Diagram to show dacryocystorhinostomy. The rhinostomy anastomoses the lacrimal sac directly to nasal mucosa, by-passing the blocked nasolacrimal duct. This operation must always be followed by a careful pharyngeal toilet to remove blood clot.

diagrammatically in Fig. 6.2. This anastomosis is lined by mucosal flaps constructed from the sac and nasal mucosal lining. The operation can be done under local anaesthesia but many patients dislike the noise of the bone-work and find it difficult to tolerate the blood running into the pharynx.

The operation is performed through an incision on the side of the nose near the medial canthus. This incision is close to and parallel with a large vein—the angular vein. Although this vein can be seen through the skin in most people, it or its tributaries are a frequent cause of copious bleeding during the operation. It avails not at all to use vasoconstrictors or arterial hypotension to staunch this flood, which may persist throughout the procedure. It is helped, to some extent, by positioning the patient in a head-up posture and by traction sutures or retractors used by the surgeon. There is a theoretical hazard of air embolism if spontaneous ventilation is used in the head-up position, but this vein usually remains full and no cases are known to have been reported. Nevertheless, it is prudent to use artificial ventilation during the operation.

Techniques
Although time consuming, there is some advantage to be gained from packing the nose with a vasoconstrictor such as cocaine paste, adrenaline or an α-adrenergic agent such as methoxamine. These can be applied on a cotton-bud jammed up the nasal bone anteriorly parallel with the bridge, or on ribbon gauze carefully packed high up on the nose. This procedure is frequently rendered difficult by a deviated septum, large turbinates and a lack of technical expertise by the anaesthetist armed with a Thudicum's nasal speculum, a head light and a pair of Tilley–Hankel

nasal packing forceps. Older techniques such as Moffat's technique of posturing the patient to ensure that cocaine, adrenaline and bicarbonate solution reach the nose have not been widely accepted in eye hospitals and probably correctly, as the vasoconstrictive effect may have worn off during the preliminary part of the operation and the construction of the bony rhinostomy.

The infiltration of a vasoconstrictor substance from the medial end of the eyebrow under the skin, down to the medial canthus and under the periosteum of the nasal bone produces a situation where the nasal bone is situated in a sandwich of vasoconstrictor agent. The technique is useful but tends to obscure the local anatomy, is quite likely to lead to intravascular injection into the angular vein, and may cause cardiac arrhythmias depending on the inhalational agent and vasoconstrictor employed. The use of adrenaline can be made safer by the concomitant administration of a beta-blocker in most patients. Methoxamine is safer but the usual intravenous preparation (20 mg/ml) needs diluting at least five times to avoid causing hypertension.

Many surgeons are capable of completing the operation within an hour before the vasoconstrictor action wears off.

Overall, the best all-round technique seems to be a combination of posture (20° head-up tilt), IPPV with some hyperventilation, and a modest reduction of blood pressure by the use of halothane.

With this method, a good field is obtained and the blood loss does not warrant replacement. It is imperative that the blood pressure should be continuously monitored throughout the procedure. Major haemorrhage is rare during operation but may occur at any time up to seven days postoperatively. Prudence dictates that the blood group of the patient is ascertained and serum stored for possible cross-matching of blood.

Canaliculo-dacryo-cysto-rhinostomy (CDCR)

A canaliculo-dacryo-cysto-rhinostomy resembles in every way the DCR already described but the emphasis is on restoring the continuity of the lacrimal canaliculi which have been interrupted by injury or disease. The surgeon uses a microscope to identify the canaliculi in relation to the medial canthal ligament. The operation is lengthy and in suitable cases controlled hypotension to a systolic pressure of 60 mmHg may be justified.

At the conclusion of all lacrimal operations, the pharynx must be checked to ensure the removal of any pack, and careful suction under direct vision must be carried out to ensure that there is no clot in the nasopharynx behind the soft palate.

Orbital surgery

The orbit is of interest not only to the ophthalmologist but also to the neurosurgeon, the rhinologist and the maxillofacial or plastic surgeon.

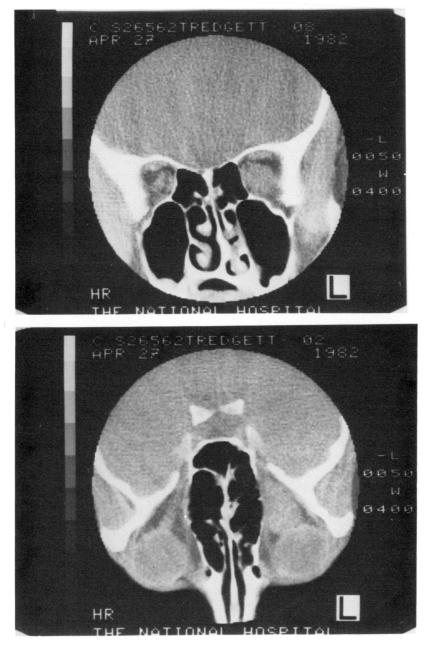

Fig. 6.3 A CT scan of an orbital tumour. This CT scan demonstrates a tumour of the left orbital nerve which has enlarged the optic canal. The right side is normal and shows the close proximity of the nasal sinuses and the extraocular muscles.

The orbital contents are not easy to expose for examination, and computerized tomography has made a major difference to the localization of orbital structures and diagnosis. (An abnormal CT scan in Fig. 6.3 shows a large tumour.) Straight radiography, angiography and ultrasound are also frequently employed.

The complexity of small structures renders delicate dissection imperative to reduce the incidence of functional and cosmetic postoperative disability. Orbital surgery tends to take place at few centres and experience of anaesthetists outside these units is very limited. Although the incidence of orbital tumour is only five per million of the population per year there is a rich variety of pathology.

Neoplasms, both primary and secondary, vascular malformations (such as the orbital varix in Fig. 6.4), dermoid cysts, acute and granulomatous inflammations, parasites, foreign bodies, fractures and endocrinopathies provide a wide range of problems and it is important that the anaesthetist should feel he is part of the surgical team and take an interest in the investigation, diagnosis, management and general care of the patients.

Orbitotomy

Anterior approach
The access to the orbit through the orbital septum anteriorly is limited as the globe fills the orbit. It is possible to take some biopsies and to remove some dermoid cysts via this route. An orbital neuroma such as that in Fig. 6.5 can be debulked by this approach. On the whole it is not possible to gain access behind the globe, although a very limited inspection of the optic nerve can be made by detaching the insertion of the medial rectus muscle and rotating the eye laterally. The major orbital operation performed anteriorly is exenteration. In the classical operation, the orbit is cleared extra-periosteally. For anteriorly placed tumours a less radical approach is used, often excising lids, conjunctival sac and enucleating the globe using cutting diathermy, Closure is by using split eyelid skin, split skin graft or by packing and allowing granulation to occur. Bleeding during anterior orbitotomy and exenteration is usually minimal and can be controlled by packs.

Lateral orbitotomy
This approach, by removal of the lateral orbital wall, allows access to all the orbital contents posterior to the globe as well as the lacrimal gland. Tumours of the lacrimal gland are an important part of an orbital surgeon's work and such a tumour is shown in Fig. 6.6. The differentiation between different orbital tissues and structures may require the use of an operating microscope and a dry field is essential. It is in this situation that profound hypotension to a systolic pressure of 60 mmHg is most rewarding. Venous bleeding is controlled by posture

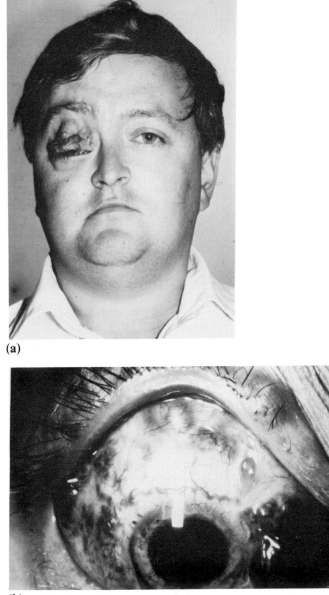

(a)

(b)

Fig. 6.4 (a) A patient with an orbital varix. This patient's orbital varices were injected with hot, hypertonic saline. Subsequent hypopituitarism led to extreme shortness of stature. Recently he has had varices resected under general anaesthesia without either blood transfusion or hormone replacement therapy. (b) An orbital varix.

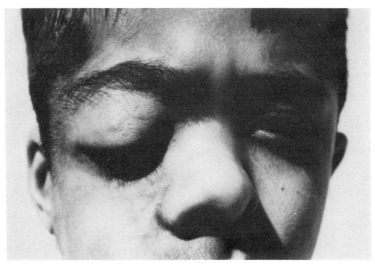

Fig. 6.5 This plexiform neuroma is an ophthalmic manifestation of neurofibromatosis in which every nerve is increased tenfold in diameter.

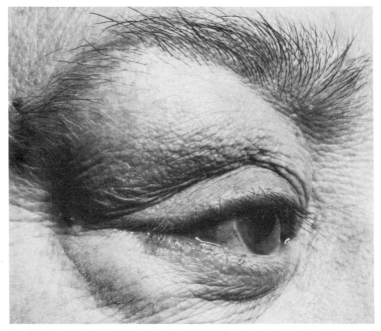

Fig. 6.6 This patient has a mixed cell tumour of the lacrimal gland. Although it appears possible to approach this anteriorly, it is not surgically practical and the tumour was removed by a lateral orbitotomy with the entire gland and the overlying periosteum.

and traction sutures, care being taken that in the head-up position air embolism is prevented by maintaining a small degree of positive intrathoracic pressure, preventing spontaneous respiration and making sure that the central venous pressure is maintained by adequate infusion.

The IOP is reduced to atmospheric and some hypotony of the globe increases the room in the orbit. Care must be taken not to compress the globe with retractors for more than a few minutes at a time as retinal ischaemia may result.

Orbital decompression

Thyroid eye disease may produce such exposure of the cornea that a keratitis is caused with corneal ulceration and oedema. However, the most serious loss of vision occurs from pressure of the orbital contents on the optic nerve. This constitutes a surgical emergency. A patient with a severe degree of thyroid disease is shown in Fig. 6.7.

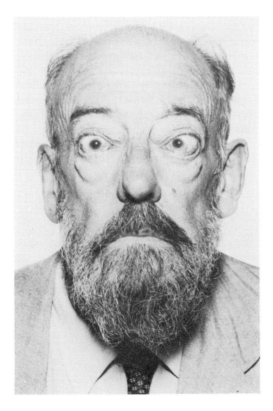

Fig. 6.7 Thyroid eye disease. This patient is likely to require a decompression of the orbit and a very careful assessment of his thyroid status by the anaesthetist.

The anaesthetic approach to these patients must always be cautious and the help of a good endocrinologist is invaluable. Apart from the management of the thyroid condition, the eye surgeons have often started treatment with massive doses of guanethidine into the conjunctival sac and systemic steroids.

The thyrotoxic patient is sometimes controlled on carbimazole and β-blockers which act for only a few hours, medication must continue up to the time of premedication to prevent 'escape' of the disease. Patients who are severely out of control may need intravenous Lugol's iodine. Although rare, the author has had one patient develop a thyrotoxic crisis under anaesthesia.

Myxoedematous patients are more common and apart from careful monitoring, particularly of core temperature, there is little that the anaesthetist can do in the short time available except minimize the dose of all drugs employed.

Vascular tumours

Although vascular tumours in the orbit are common, severe haemorrhage is rare. Orbital varices of enormous size are really stagnant venous lakes; cavernous haemangiomata are well encapsulated and shell out with careful dissection. The problems tend to arise in the arteriovenous fistulae which lead to pulsating exophthalmos. The fistulae are usually multiple and may involve bone. Sometimes the arterial connection is with the carotid artery in the cavernous sinus. These tumours require adequate facilities for transfusion and a lot of cross-matched blood. As surgery is usually only palliative, the surgeon may need to be warned of the dangers to the patient, lest his enthusiasm encourages him to a disaster.

Further reading

Edridge, A. (1963). Anaesthetic aspects of hypotension in eye surgery. *Proceedings of Royal Society of Medicine* **56**, 985.

Smith, G.B. (1973). Anaesthesia for lacrimal surgery. *Transactions of the Ophthalmological Societies of the UK* **93**, 619.

Smith, G.B. (1979). Anaesthetic techniques for orbital surgery. *Transactions of the Ophthalmological Societies of the UK* **99**, 236.

Smith, G.B. (1975). Anaesthesia for orbital surgery. *Modern Problems in Ophthalmology* **14**, 457.

7

Paediatric anaesthesia in eye surgery

In Britain, children are treated in adult eye units at hospitals, whereas, in some other countries, paediatric ophthalmic units are part of children's hospitals. This leads to some difference in emphasis and anaesthetic management. The children's ward in an eye hospital needs to be a happy, active place with specialist children's nurses and the frequent presence of a paediatrician. Separate accommodation is required for infants and for children. The children on such a ward may be blind or partially sighted but are seldom ill. Indeed, a child who is ill should not be there. This system means that much of the infrastructure of a children's hospital may be lacking but must be provided in an adjacent paediatric unit. To illustrate this situation let us imagine the problems of assessing the retinal functions of a six-month-old Negro baby with homozygous sickle cell disease. The baby can or should be admitted with the mother. Skilled children's nursing and feeding will present no problem. The assessment of the general condition can be made on one of the paediatrician's regular visits to the eye hospital. Special haematological investigations will be required on small blood samples. The anaesthetist will make a preoperative visit to arrange premedication and to make his own assessment of the situation. The child is prepared for theatre and eventually is sent for. Adult ophthalmic units do not usually allow parents into the theatre accommodation. There is, in the anaesthetic room, a limited amount of paediatric equipment; a mask, a laryngoscope and a tube of suitable size are easily found. A heating blanket, rectal thermometer, precordial (or oesophageal) stethoscope and paediatric blood-pressure cuff are necessary. Scalp vein needles, paediatric infusion sets, infant ventilators and suitable monitoring leads are not usually available in eye hospitals and there are distinct difficulties in obtaining adequate humidification of inspired gases or blood-gas analysis. Should the child be unwell postoperatively, then it is transferred to the nearby children's hospital where there is round-the-clock cover by paediatricians.

This exaggeration of the problems of paediatric anaesthesia in an eye hospital highlights the difficulties and ignores the excellent record in most eye hospitals where extremely skilled anaesthetists manage with great skill and minimal facilities to perform a difficult task with safety on very large numbers of children of all ages, amounting to about one-fifth of the total anaesthetics given.

The most common eye condition among children is strabismus, accounting for about two-thirds of children having surgery under general anaesthesia. The remaining one-third is made up of congenital cataract, ptosis, trauma, lacrimal diseases and a considerable number of diagnostic examinations under anaesthesia. Rare conditions such as retinoblastoma inside the globe, rhabdomyosarcoma and dermoid cyst in the orbit and angiomatous conditions of the lids tend to find their way to highly specialized national hospitals. Congenital glaucoma is an important but rare cause of blindness among children; other congenital defects are too numerous to mention here and the reader is referred to Harley's (1975) excellent book on *Pediatric Ophthalmology*.

Anaesthesia for examination and for congenital cataract

The anaesthetist should beware of the child with one defect because in many children defects tend to be multiple and sometimes there is also an additional inborn error of metabolism. Some examples are given below.

Airway problems

The Pierre Robin syndrome of micrognathia and cleft palate may be associated with congenital cataract or congenital glaucoma. Babies with Treacher Collins syndrome of micrognathia, high arched palate with clefts of lip or palate may have coloboma, microphthalmos and anti-mongoloid slant.

Metabolic problems

Glycogen storage disease and phenylketonuria may both cause severe hypoglycaemia on starvation. Both are associated with congenital cataract, as are many of the diseases of amino acid metabolism.

Neurological problems

Dystrophia myotonica, myasthenia gravis, acute porphyria and familial dysautonomia present rare but recurring problems because of their association with squints.

The most disastrous condition is irreversible malignant hyperpyrexia which may occur in any child but particularly those having strabismus surgery. The triggering drug in most patients seems to be suxamethonium followed by halothane, the combination of the two being particularly dangerous in this rare condition. It is a general rule among the author's colleagues to intubate all children using inhalational agents only (usually halothane). The incidence of malignant hyperpyrexia seems to be low. Our only proven case in over 80 000 anaesthetics recovered completely after a rapid diagnosis, termination of anaesthesia and bicarbonate infusion.

Strabismus

There is an increasing tendency for surgeons to undertake eye muscle surgery between 6 and 12 months of age to allow the squinting eye to develop normal vision and in the hope of allowing the two eyes to acquire stereopsis. However, many older children do not have their squints corrected until school entry or later.

The older children need careful handling on the preanaesthetic visit as they can seldom appreciate the value of the surgery and it is better for them to view the anaesthetist as a friend rather than as a stranger. This is particularly important as the ideal premedicant has yet to be devised.

Younger children are premedicated with trimeprazine 6 mg/kg with atropine 10 μg/kg by mouth. Oral atropine seems to be generally effective in controlling secretions and reducing bradycardia. Older children may be given papaveretum and hyoscine parenterally or diazepam 0.1 mg/kg.

We practise inhalational anaesthesia with nitrous oxide–oxygen–halothane on most children to the age of 6 or 7 and then use an adult-type of induction technique. Cyclopropane is seldom used nowadays for induction. The usual techniques are used for intubation, maintenance and monitoring. It is worthwhile supporting the child's head in a ring or grommet to prevent movement during surgery. Many children have flexion of the cervical spine when lying on a flat surface; this impedes surgical access and the shoulders need raising on a 4 cm pad to bring the face into a horizontal position.

Tension on the recti during surgery may cause cardiac slowing and if this is severe, atropine 10 mg/kg may be injected.

Congenital cataract

A careful history and examination may show the cause of the cataract and indicate its relevance to anaesthesia. It is interesting that cataracts caused by maternal rubella during pregnancy may harbour the virus for the first few years of life, and direct contact with any fluid from the eye should be avoided.

The surgeon will generally incise the lens capsule through the dilated pupil and aspirate the lens matter through an irrigating cannula.

Ptosis

This is rarely symptomatic of myasthenia gravis in children but usually results from congenital or hereditary disease of the third nerve. It is seldom necessary to perform a Tensilon (edrophonium) test below the age of 10 years unless the ptosis is of fluctuating degree.

Retinoblastoma

This may present sporadically at any age but often in children and in one eye. The tumour is, however, inheritable by dominant genes with partial penetrance, and in children in whom there is a family history it may even occur *in utero* and tends to be multifocal and bilateral. The anaesthetic problem is the repeated examination under anaesthesia of children or relatives of a known case from the first week of life onwards, initially monthly and then at longer intervals up to the age of 6 years.

The frequency of these examinations presents problems of a psychological nature to the child and is a challenge to the anaesthetist in terms of premedication and induction. Ideally, the same anaesthetist should continue to look after the child throughout the first years of life. Trimeprazine premedication is often recognized and rejected by the child and resort to parenteral premedication is found to be necessary. Ample well-trained assistance is needed in the anaesthetic room, particularly as the children get larger and more rebellious, but if the child has time to settle down or can be induced into going to sleep naturally, a smooth induction is often obtained.

Because these tumours often start peripherally in the retina, the surgeon requires a well-dilated pupil and needs to indent the outside of the eye—this produces strong stimulation and requires a fairly deep plane of anaesthesia. Ketamine has not proved very satisfactory in the usually recommended dosage. An insufflation technique may be adequate for the smaller child but if photocoagulation, cryotherapy or application of a cobalt plaque is required, then full endotracheal anaesthesia is essential. Large tumours involving the optic disc are usually referred to major centres and if the diagnosis is confirmed, the eye is enucleated with a length of optic nerve.

Congenital glaucoma

Most cases present at birth or during the first year of life. Some are associated with the Sturge–Weber syndrome in which angiomata may affect the face, body, mouth and larynx. The presenting signs are a baby with photophobia with large, cloudy corneas. Frequently the disease is bilateral.

The surgeon will wish to examine the child at frequent intervals to measure the corneal diameter, check the intraocular pressure, examine the cupping of the optic disc and look at the drainage angle of the anterior chamber. The examination takes about 30 minutes.

The definitive treatment of this condition is the production of a cleft in the drainage angle by a fine knife passed across the anterior chamber from a stab incision. This goniotomy allows drainage of aqueous humour and arrests the condition. It is very rapid, takes place down a microscope but needs the head to be perfectly still during the operation. It is another procedure in which ketamine is not suitable.

The special anaesthetic problem of these children is to obtain accurate reproducible readings of intraocular pressure to demonstrate the satisfactory response to treatment and the containment of the disease. Until recently, ether was the method of choice for the first part of the examination under anaesthesia, then changing to halothane which lowered the intraocular pressure and allowed clearing of any corneal oedema.

Since 1976, Coren has been using a technique based on intramuscular ketamine 6–10 mg/kg. Only if goniotomy is required is this followed by intubation and very light halothane anaesthesia. The transition from ketamine to halothane is not always easy in small babies and special experience of this technique is required.

Paediatric ophthalmic anaesthesia is perhaps a specialty in itself.

References

Coren, A. Personal communication.
Harley, R.D. (1975). *Pediatric Ophthalmology*. W.B. Sanders, Philadelphia.

8

Oculocardiac reflex, eyedrops and monitoring

Oculocardiac reflex

It was in 1908 that Aschner observed that application of pressure to the eyeball caused a reduction in the pulse rate. It is interesting that this first observation is often ignored and more attention is paid to traction on the extraocular muscles than to raised intraocular pressure. In fact, the reflex can be triggered by a number of stretch and pressure stimuli in the orbit and produces a variety of physiological results which may lead to errors in diagnosis.

The pain and increased pressure of acute glaucoma are associated with abdominal distress and vomiting. It is not always appreciated that intraocular pressure frequently rises in the postoperative period to reach those values found in acute glaucoma; thus the patient whose cataract was removed through a corneal section, which has been perfectly repaired by a continuous 10/0 suture, will sometimes feel nauseated or actually vomit 24 hours postoperatively, not because he has had an opiate, nor because of delayed effects of general anaesthesia, not even because of impaired hepatic function, but simply on account of very accurate surgery and suturing which has left the globe so watertight that there is no accommodation for any inflammatory results inside the eye; the pressure rises and pain with vomiting ensue. The treatment of such a case is to be alert to this situation and, providing the ophthalmic surgeon is in agreement, to add acetazolamide to any anti-emetics or analgesics and thereby help to lower the intraocular pressure. It may be pharmacologically correct to attempt to block the vagal impulses with atropine but atropine and its congeners are more effective on the cardiac vagus than on the abdominal viscera.

Nearly every procedure for retinal detachment includes scleral buckling by plombage or silastic strap, as shown in Fig. 8.1. If the retinal hole remains open, then the eye tends to remain hypotonic but, once this is sealed, the pressure rapidly rises. Length of anaesthesia or the pain of incision is blamed for postoperative nausea but the true cause is pressure pain. It is difficult to examine the eyes of these patients postoperatively because of intense blepharospasm, but in the presence of a bradycardia it is reasonable to assume the tension is raised and treatment should once

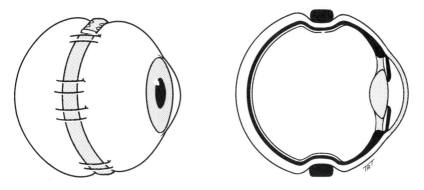

Fig. 8.1 'Encirclement' of the globe using a silicone rubber band is a procedure often used to buckle the sclera during vitreous or detachment surgery. It can be easily seen how this operation can activate the oculocardiac reflex, particularly if fluid is not drained from inside the eye.

again include measures to reduce the pressure as well as anti-emetics and analgesics.

The presence of the globe is not necessary for this reflex. On several occasions, a disproportionate amount of shock has followed a small postoperative haemorrhage after enucleation of the eyeball.

One particular patient, when returned to the ward, became so pale, sweaty, nauseated and hypotensive that eminent cardiologists diagnosed postoperative myocardial infarction; the true diagnosis was only revealed when removal of the eye pad and bandage disclosed a small haematoma. This patient showed a bradycardia with many irregularities.

The neurological pathway

The reflex is transmitted by the trigeminal nerve to the main sensory nucleus of V. It is blocked by local anaesthesia of the fifth nerve and by retrobulbar injection of anaesthetic. The efferent pathway is by the vagus nerve and the cardiac effects may be blocked by atropine, gallamine and glycopyrrolate.

Incidence

The most common presentation of the oculocardiac reflex is when traction is applied to the extraocular muscles. Alexander (1975) recorded this occurrence in 90 per cent of patients. Most patients have a bradycardia which may halve the pulse rate; in a few, junctional rhythm or bigeminal rhythm occurs. Apt *et al.* (1973) noticed that the medial rectus is much more sensitive than the lateral rectus. It is important that the same degree of tension is applied when comparing the response of individual muscles to a stretch stimulus.

Because of the frequency with which this reflex occurs, it is important to consider the danger to the patient. It is surprising and very significant that at Moorfields Eye Hospital during the last 15 years, in which approximately 100 000 operations were done under general anaesthesia, there have been no deaths attributable to this reflex. Improving standards of anaesthesia, increased awareness of the reflex and better monitoring have obviously had a part to play in this situation—even so, the reflex itself must be fairly benign and many of the recorded deaths in the past may have been the result of kinking of the endotracheal tube, the exhaustion of an oxygen cylinder or other anaesthetic accidents such as malignant hyperpyrexia or gastric aspiration. In brief, it would be safe to say that the oculocardiac reflex occurs frequently, but seldom, if ever, kills.

Prophylaxis and treatment

It is arguable whether it is worthwhile to give the massive doses of atropine required to block the vagus. The usual premedicant dose of atropine (0.01 mg/kg) is in the region of one-fifth of that required to block the vagus but is probably sufficient to reduce the degree of cardiac slowing and inhibit the occurrence of arrhythmias. Oral atropine is very useful in children undergoing strabismus surgery and atropine is added to the trimeprazine syrup used as a premedicant.

Premedicant syrup:
   trimeprazine 6 mg/ml
   atropine 0.05 mg/ml
   dose 0.5–0.75 ml/kg by mouth.

This seems successful in drying the secretions and blocking the reflex up to 6 years of age. It is not always a reliable sedative but seems remarkably safe.

In older children and adults, atropine may be given intramuscularly but there is an increasing tendency to use diazepam or lorazepam orally and the anaesthetist gives atropine intravenously at the time of induction. There has been much published on the possible arrhythmias likely to be caused by intravenous atropine but, once again, although real, they are benign and short lived. The antisialogogue actions of atropine are less marked with the intravenous route and the dose often needs increasing to 1 mg or more in the average adult.

During operation or in recovery, the pulse rate may fall to 40 beats/minute and it is not established whether it is desirable to treat bradycardia with intravenous atropine or to adopt a wait-and-see attitude. It is very seldom that the bradycardia become sufficiently severe to cause circulatory insufficiency.

There seems to be no indication for the use of hyoscine (scopolamine) in ophthalmic surgery as its long action and tendency to cause postoperative confusion become more apparent when the policy is one of early ambulation. The latest parasympatholytic agent—glycopyrrolate—has not been available long enough nor has it been used sufficiently extensively to warrant expressing an opinion on its place in this form of anaesthesia.

Eyedrops

The conjunctiva is a waterproof layer which absorbs drugs slowly, if at all. It is much more impervious than the thinner epithelium that covers the cornea. Thus, drops instilled into the conjunctival sac tend to have an action on the eye but little systemic action. In the conscious patient, drugs are carried through the lacrimal apparatus to the nose where the nasal mucosa absorbs them rapidly to produce systemic effects. The lacrimal apparatus depends for its efficient action on the blink reflex and muscle action. When these become inoperative during general anaesthesia, then little is absorbed into the bloodstream. This is fortunate as many eyedrops are extremely powerful agents in massive concentration. The red or inflamed eye may encourage the surgeon to ask the anaesthetist whether it is safe to instil a vasoconstrictor such as adrenaline. There is little evidence that drugs are absorbed any faster in most of these eyes providing the conjunctiva remains intact. Eye surgeons are sometimes surprised that their drops can cause systemic effects.

Gutt adrenaline

This is labelled as 1:1000 and 1:10 000 but ophthalmic adrenaline is poor stuff as it is dispensed as a neutral solution which is very unstable and despite refrigeration has only weak vasoconstrictor properties. In the conscious patient it is frequently given as regular medication in the control of glaucoma. The control of intraocular pressure is only obtained at the cost of producing a chronically congested conjunctiva. In the unconscious patient, the surgeon may request an adrenaline drop to improve haemostasis and some surgeons regard this as a routine. Rarely, a few extrasystoles are induced some minutes after the instillation but the author has yet to hear of ventricular fibrillation being induced in a young patient who has been given adrenaline drops when receiving the vapour of a halogenated hydrocarbon such as halothane or trichlorethylene. The nervous anaesthetist might consider giving the patient an adrenergic beta-blocker to reduce cardiac irregularities. Adrenaline drops are weak dilators of the pupil.

Gutt phenylephrine 10 per cent

This drug was first used as a pressor agent in spinal anaesthesia. It is an alpha-simulator and also causes direct constriction of vessel walls. There is little effect on bronchial musculature nor is there a cerebral stimulant action. It is a very powerful dilator of the pupil but causes some damage to corneal endothelium.

When it is given before induction of anaesthesia it causes contraction of Müller's muscle and the cornea may be exposed once general anaesthesia has been induced.

Because of its effectiveness, it is sometimes instilled into the eyes of babies prior to an examination under anaesthesia. This causes gross tachycardia and hypertension. When required in children it should be given very sparingly and atropine substituted where possible.

Atropine 1 per cent or 2 per cent

Some patients are surprisingly sensitive to this drug. As one drop of 1% atropine contains 2 mg or 3 mg of atropine and if absorption from the nasal mucosa is complete, then it is not unexpected that patients written up for twice-daily atropine exhibit some degree of belladonna poisoning. In children, this takes the form of pyrexia and scarletiniform skin rashes, while in adults tachycardia is the presenting feature. The pyrexia in children is frequently misdiagnosed and causes postponement of operation.

Localized sensitivity is a problem but this should not prevent atropine being used parenterally, for example in premedication.

Ecothiopate (phospholine iodide)

Several concentrations of this drug are used in the control of glaucoma. It is an organophosphorous compound related to the insecticides and nerve gases. It is absorbed from the conjunctival sac and depletes serum cholinesterase for up to three weeks from the last dose. When possible, it is desirable that it should be discontinued for three weeks prior to planned surgery. There have been exaggerated reports of the severity of the apnoea which may follow the use of suxamethonium. The apnoea usually lasts twice or three times the normal length of time and can be minimized by reducing the dose of suxamethonium. It may often be cautious to substitute a non-depolarizing muscle relaxant; however, when this is done, the relaxation is less than expected.

Mydricaine

Prolonged surgery on the posterior segment of the eye and the insertion of lens implants into the posterior chamber require an intense mydriasis which may not be achieved very easily with eyedrops, particularly if the iris is heavily pigmented. The ophthalmic surgeons have re-discovered the value of preparations whose original purpose may have been different. At Moorfields Eye Hospital there has been a considerable increase in the use of the subconjunctival injection of 'Mydricaine'. This is a mydriatic of enormous potency originally formulated to break down adhesions or synechiae between the iris and the lens as the result of uveitis.

Mydricaine No. 1 has the formula:
procaine hydrochloride 3 mg
atropine sulphate 500 mcg
boric acid 5 mg
adrenaline 1/1000 0.06 ml
sodium meta-bisulphite 0.1% w/v
water for injection 0.3 ml
total volume 0.5 ml
Mydricaine No. 2 has twice the concentration of the active constituents in the same volume.

The injection of this dose of adrenaline may lead to tachycardia and ectopic cardiac rhythms, particularly in a myocardium sensitized to adrenaline by halogenated volatile agents. This effect is transient and may be abolished by β-adrenergic blockade.

Monitoring

Ophthalmic anaesthesia tends to take place on very young or very old patients. Once the operation has started there is very poor access to the airway, which must be impeccable from the outset.

Frequently the theatre lights are dimmed or extinguished. It is very important that the anaesthetist should be satisfied with the ventilation of the patient, whether it is spontaneous or controlled. It is desirable that the anaesthetist can measure expired minute volumes and probably end-tidal carbon dioxide concentrations. These demonstrate the integrity of the airway and the efficiency of ventilation. The electrocardiographic monitor demonstrates the rhythm and electrical activity of the heart and all modern versions incorporate alarm systems.

The blood pressure should be measured at intervals by oscillo-tonometry if an automated system is not available.

More complex monitoring than this is not economic for procedures lasting an hour or less, particularly as there is little metabolic disturbance or blood loss in ophthalmic work. Diabetic patients will need hourly blood-sugar estimations.

In longer operations, particularly on the elderly who have been taking diuretics for years, inadequate reversal of relaxants becomes a problem in the presence of total body potassium depletion. Similar problems may arise in myasthenia gravis and various muscular dystrophies. It is helpful to assess the benefit of therapeutic measures with a peripheral nerve stimulator capable of producing train-of-four supramaximal nerve stimuli.

References

Alexander, J.P. (1975). Reflex disturbance of cardiac rhythm during ophthalmic surgery. *British Journal of Ophthalmology* **59**, 518.
Aschner, S. (1908). Uber einen bisher nochnicht beschriebenen Reflex von Auge auf Kreislauf und Atmung. *Weiner Klinische Wochenshrift* **21**, 1529.
Apt, C., Isebnerg, S. and Gaffney, W.L. (1973). The oculocardiac reflex in strabismus surgery. *American Journal of Ophthalmology* **76**, 533.

9

Mortality in ophthalmic anaesthesia

Incidence

The increasing average age of patients in North America and Europe combined with improved facilities for and use of general anaesthesia in ophthalmic units, render data, such as that in Table 9.1, collected as recently as ten years ago, obsolete. There are, however, certain trends which are reflected in mortality figures and some relevant conclusions to be drawn.

Duncalf *et al.* (1970) collected the figures for 197 653 patients in North America in 1967, but this represented a selected sample because this poll included the records of only 16 per cent of the ophthalmic surgeons in the country.

Of these patients, 70 744 had general anaesthesia with a mortality of 0.65/1000 compared with the remainder who has a mortality of 0.62/1000 under local anaesthesia. It is essential to interpret these figures with caution as the two groups of patients were unlikely to have been homogeneous, the cases selected for local anaesthesia usually having a high average age and often a shorter procedure such as a cataract extraction, while the operations under general anaesthesia must have included many children and middle-aged patients with retinal detachments.

Kaplan and Reber (1972) emphasized the importance of autopsy in

Table 9.1 Mortality of anaesthesia in ophthalmic surgery

			Deaths/1000		
		Patients	GA	LA	Overall
Duncalf	(1967)	197 653	0.65	0.62	0.63
Kaplan	(1958–70)	21 400			1.40
Petruscak	(1962–71)	31 322	0.35	0.69	0.51
Quigley	(1952–72)	47 000	1.17	1.50	1.60*
Hallermann	(1963–74)	11 000	1.64	1.62	1.63

*This includes 12 patients who died without anaesthesia or operation.

 This table demonstrates an overall mortality for up to 20 days or more postoperatively and Quigley had no deaths in the operating theatre or recovery room in the second part of his series totalling 17 155 patients, of whom exactly half had general anaesthesia.

determining the cause of death as, in the presence of multiple pathology in elderly patients, errors in diagnosis were frequent. They were surprised to find that with a post-mortem rate of 63 per cent, 9 of 19 autopsies showed that pulmonary embolism was the cause of death in spite of the fact that most patients were ambulatory within 24 hours of operation.

This confirmed the earlier figures of Kristensen (1966) that the average time of death following cataract extraction is on the eleventh day, and underlines the fact that a long period of postoperative surveillance is required to obtain true figures and that in eye hospitals, where the length of stay may be as short as five days, it is not possible to obtain meaningful figures.

Unfortunately, Kaplan and Reber do not record how many of their 21 400 patients received general anaesthesia, but of the 30 recorded deaths in their series, 19 occurred following the administration of local anaesthesia. Because they followed up their patients for 20 days, their overall mortality reached the figure of 1.4 deaths/1000. It is interesting to note that their series started in 1960 and the median age of death was 75 years.

Reporting from Baltimore in 1974, Quigley reached similar conclusions from 47 000 operations. His figures are interesting as they include four patients who died without anaesthesia or surgery and a further eight patients who died after transfer to another hospital because they were too ill for any procedure to be performed. It is remarkable that he provides figures suggesting that, in his city, patients wih a lower socio-economic background have twice the chance of dying as the result of ophthalmic surgery. He claims a mortality rate of 1.6 deaths/1000 and, of the cases coming to autopsy, 9 out of 32 died from pulmonary embolism, 6 from myocardial infarction and 6 from cerebrovascular accident. One patient died of liver failure following two general anaesthetics for retinal detachment which lasted a total of 9.5 hours. This would be in agreement with several deaths at Moorfields Eye Hospital which have been labelled 'halothane' hepatitis!

Petruscak et al. (1973) from Pittsburgh reported no mortality in 17 155 operations over a five-year span in the operating room or recovery room, although six patients who received local anaesthesia and three patients who received general anaesthesia died postoperatively within 20 days.

They attribute this low rate to better patient care, improved preoperative assessment and investigation of patients, and monitoring both during operation and in the postoperative recovery room.

Experience in Germany is similar to that in the United States. Hallermann and Ruger (1976) were using either general or neuroleptic techniques in 90 per cent of their operations. In 11 000 operations over the preceding period, they achieved a mortality rate of 1.63 deaths/1000 for general anaesthesia (GA) and 1.64 deaths/1000 for local anaesthesia

(LA). Pulmonary embolism was twice as likely to occur after local anaesthesia, while cardiac and hepatic problems were more common when general anaesthesia was used.

British figures are difficult to obtain because the major eye hospitals tend to be detached from the general hospital to whose respiratory, cardiac, hepatic and renal units complicated postoperative problems are referred. The difficulties in communication tend to render statistics incomplete.

The study of Mortality Associated with Anaesthesia (Lunn and Mushin, 1982), investigating 6060 deaths based on over one million operations, will be a landmark for British anaesthetists for many years to come. Its conclusions on preoperative assessment, preoxygenation, the use of monitoring equipment and the maintenance of anaesthetic records are among the foundations of good anaesthetic practice and will be taken seriously by all anaesthetists including those working in eye hospitals.

Unfortunately, the response rate of 61 per cent to questionnaires, the inadequacy of the records supplied and reliance on the subjective opinions of assessors render the validity of some of the figures open to question, although they reveal interesting trends in current practice. There are no overall mortality figures for ophthalmology. However, in the 59 deaths in which anaesthesia was held to be totally responsible, there were 2 deaths recorded of patients undergoing bilateral cataract extractions. In only one of these are further details provided. This patient was a 79-year-old diabetic woman who sustained a cardiac arrest 15 minutes after induction of anaesthesia. It is suggested in this report that oesophageal intubation or autonomic neuropathy may have played some part. It is to be hoped that future surveys of this type may elucidate the problems more precisely so that remedies may be sought and applied.

References

Duncalf, D., Gartner, S. and Carol, B. (1970). Mortality in association with ophthalmic surgery. *American Journal of Ophthalmology* **69**, 610.

Hallermann, W. and Ruger, J. (1976). Zwischenfälle und Letalität bei Augenoperationer. *Klinishe Monatsblaetter für Augenheilkunde* **169**, 700.

Kaplan, M.R. and Reber, R.C. (1972). Pulmonary embolism as the leading cause of ophthalmic mortality. *American Journal of Ophthalmology* **73**, 159.

Lunn, J.N. and Mushin, W.W (1982). *Mortality Associated with Anaesthetics*. Nuffield Provincial Hospitals Trust.

Petruscak, J., Smith, R.B. and Breslin, P. (1973). Mortality related to ophthalmological surgery. *Archives of Ophthalmology* **89**, 106.

Quigley, H.A. (1974). Mortality associated with ophthalmic surgery. *American Journal of Ophthalmology* **77**, 517.

Index